ATRIAL FRUSTRATION

ATRIAL FRUSTRATION

A Cardiac Arrhythmia Saga

Adam C. Ehlert

Cover design by Janelle Smith, Smith Visual Communication Arts.

Photos by Heather Ehlert.

To my pretty girls: Heather and Moxie.

Thank you for your love and support.

And with special appreciation for
all medical professionals.

Your kind patience tempers your impatient patients.

CONTENTS

FOREWORD

Atrial Fibrillation (AF) is an arrhythmia due to irregular and chaotic electrical activity within the atrium. It is the most prevalent arrhythmia worldwide, affecting 1.5-6% of the population, with numbers anticipated to double over the next decade. It is also the leading cause of stroke. With the aging population and medical comorbidities, the incidence of AF continues to rise and heading towards epidemic proportions. There has been significant progress made in the identification and treatment of AF. The pursuit of a potential cure of AF either by medications or a procedure so far has been disappointing.

The fundamental reason for this appears to be a lack of a clear understanding of the mechanism of AF. The paradigm of contemporary AF management is based on rate control, rhythm control, and stroke prevention. There have been significant strides made to define an optimum heart rate, medications to facilitate adequate rate and rhythm control, and a myriad of ablation techniques to maintain sinus rhythm. Warfarin, along with several newer oral anticoagulants, is available for stroke prevention.

As no two people look alike, everyone's AF is unique, but the treatment offered remains uniform to everyone. We realized quite early in our quest to treat AF that *"one size fits all"* mantra leads to *wardrobe malfunctions*!

There has been a tectonic shift in approaching AF from a disease of the atrium to a marker of underlying vascular health and wellness. It has resulted in aggressive measures in trying to improve health by weight loss, improving cardiopulmonary fitness, and aggressive management of comorbidities such as hypertension, sleep apnea, diabetes, among others.

With the advent of wearable technology such as smartwatches and other sensor-based technologies, patients can potentially self-diagnose AF before being seen by healthcare providers. It certainly has several advantages, but simultaneously has created unique challenges. There has been considerable personal angst in self-checking for any arrhythmias and potentially coming up with a treatment plan based on information gathered from non-peer-reviewed resources. The internet can be a useful resource, but it cannot replace a nurse or a doctor.

As a medical fraternity, we aim to alleviate the pain and suffering of the patients. However, the treatment of AF does pose a question of whether we should treat the patient, cure the electrocardiogram, or alleviate the anxiety associated with the diagnosis of AF. Beyond risk stratification for the prevention of stroke, the rest of the treatment options are intended to improve the quality of the life of the patient. It is beyond science and medicine to make a person with no symptoms feel better!

Everyone's story of life in general, and specifically of AF is different. The trigger for AF in one person, such as exercise, maybe a treatment for another person with AF to facilitate weight loss. Hence it is but natural for our patients to be concerned and confused about what exactly needs to be. This dilemma is also faced by the caregiver to identify the right and the most effective and safe treatment for a particular patient.

In this book, the author *(who truly is "a delightful young man from Kansas")* shares his journey with atrial fibrillation or atrial frustration. Many of the readers would be able to empathize with the author. I wish the author, the book, and specifically the readers the very best in their AF odyssey.

Nevertheless, remember you are not alone in this, and your doctor can and will be a great travel companion in this adventure.

Abhishek Deshmukh, MD, FHRS
Consultant Electrophysiologist
Mayo Clinic, Rochester MN

INTRODUCTION

The first thing I learned about atrial fibrillation remains the most important thing I know about atrial fibrillation.

Nearly twenty years ago as a medical student I attended a lecture about this heart rhythm abnormality and an extremely insightful physician proclaimed that it was rarely about the atrial fibrillation alone, and quite commonly about the underlying conditions that first triggered the atrial fibrillation in the beginning.

Mr. Ehlert's account of his ongoing experience is no exception – it was never just his atrial fibrillation, it was truly about a congenital heart defect, present since birth, that required repair. Yet we often focus on the arrhythmia itself and spend too little time on the potential and exceedingly important underlying triggers including high blood pressure, physical inactivity, structural heart disease, diet, sleep disorders, and body size, to name just a few. Mr. Ehlert's unique perspective and pervasive frustration has the promise to serve as a springboard for patients to think beyond their atrial fibrillation and direct equal, due attention to these important conditions.

Henry G. Riter, MD, Cardiologist

It's not a heart attack, but…

WAS IT FEAR?

Of course it was fear. Self-admitted or not. And maybe a little machismo. Why couldn't I pick up the phone? I wasn't dying. Right? So why did I need to bother? And since I was not dying, it really was no bother. But I was curious. And worried. And I wondered how I would have been able to justify *not* doing anything. I finally overcame my faux-machismo.

"Is Dr. Powers in today—might be he able to squeeze me in?"

"No, I'm afraid he's out of the office now for about three weeks."

"Okay, I'll call back when I can schedule that far ahead."

A couple of hours later I climbed my stairs again. Not a huge climb. Two flights, 24 steps total; 11 and 13, why not 12 and 12? Even with my rhythmic stair-counting distraction, I knew something was not right. But I also knew (?) it was not a heart attack, and therefore not life threatening (of course…).

"Hi, I'm a patient of Dr. Powers' and I had called earlier. I understand he's out of town, but might another physician be able to see me today?"

"What do you need, what are your symptoms, sir?"

"Well, I don't think it's a heart attack, but I feel a little funny—I'm lightheaded, especially after even very light exertion, like climbing stairs. I don't have any real pain, but it just feels like something is "off," and I really cannot catch my breath. I'm not really 'clammy,' but I am maybe sweatier than I should be on this temperate spring day. Actually, clammy might be a good word for it."

"Sir (and I know she used that word tentatively—she was a professional, trying to be respectful to the halfwit customer on the phone), I strongly recommend you go somewhere with the word 'Emergency' in its name. Are you nearby? Can I call our local hospital? It's only two miles away—or, maybe a smarter call is for an ambulance."

"Okay, thank you for your advice—I will do that. Afterwards, I will call and report what I've learned, so you can get it in my file."

I know she was practicing big-medicine CYA, but I had been walking around like this for two days; I did not need her to call an ambulance for me.

———

Reading between the nurse's lines, I inferred some assurance that I was not going to expire in the next couple hours. So, I drove home, changed clothes, brought in the mail, maybe had a snack…and then drove to the emergency room 11 minutes from my house. Sweating nervously the whole time.

I'd lived in this city for nearly ten years, but as a healthy young male, had never had occasion to use my local hospital. I knew it had a good reputation, though, and was glad this one was close, especially as rush hour was approaching.

I followed the bright red signs for EMERGENCY, and walked in the automatic doors. Even without first-hand use of real hospital-style services, I still considered myself somewhat savvy as a medical customer. But I was wondering—do they get many walk-ins here? This is prototypical suburbia, in prototypical—and literal—middle America. Not a lot of gunshot wound victims are dropped at the door, nor many overdose victims at 4:00 on a Tuesday afternoon. My dreams of appearing in the background of a COPS episode were drowsily dashed.

So, I tentatively walked in my slim-ish, six-foot self, and the clerks looked up attentively, hopeful for some action. I began recounting my story, trying to detail how

I had felt to precipitate my two calls to my regular doctor. Once I hit the meat of the matter, they moved quickly. Before I got the entire phrase "lightheaded, short of breath" out of my mouth, they had me sacked into a chair, its wheels rolling back into an examination room.

In the few years since my inaugural episode, I've of course shared my story. I recently discovered a friend has been similarly afflicted, and he's got a great description: "bingo balls and rubber mallets (bouncing around in my chest)." I love it! Granted, in another context, the symptomatic description of "bingo balls and rubber mallets" could have a markedly different connotation to the uninitiated. But, to us experienced arrhythmics, it works. For my first run-through, though, I was unable to describe my symptoms in such an illustrative manner.

From that first strap-in, I do not recall many details. It took a few hours. I didn't feel like my life was in danger, but if it was, I was in the right place. I held off on calling my wife for a while, hoping I might have a quick explanation, discharge, and would make it home for dinner. No problem, no worry.

From the outset, obviously, they knew it was heart-related. I *now* know the terms and procedures. *Then*, I had no idea. We removed my shirt and they started applying stickers and wires and attaching those wires to machines that were wheeled in expeditiously. I'm fairly certain they did not spare the two minutes (that is if the nurse does a delicate, caring job) to do any shaving of arms or chest.

My strongest detailed memory is overhearing the ER doctor on the phone (with, I now understand, a cardiologist): “It is classic AFib, but he’s way too young for that!”

After several hours, we got that official confirmation: I was suffering from a very common form of an irregular heartbeat called Atrial Fibrillation. Little did I know that this was just the camel’s nose under the tent.

I don’t recall feeling particularly concerned—they can fix anything with a pill or two, right? And I’m otherwise healthy. I suspected that once I did let my wife know my whereabouts, that they probably wouldn’t let me drive home. She always rises to the occasion, and had already scrambled for a ride *to* the hospital from our saintly neighbor so that we didn’t have to worry about retrieving a car *from* the hospital in the middle of the night...or next week, or whenever. Simple logistics can become a headache though this saga.

———

The doctor was helpful as he talked us through his diagnosis and as the cadre of nurses and techs removed me from the electrical grid and more strenuously removed the hair from my well-monitored chest and arm where the just-in-case IV had been.

They had made an appointment for me with the cardiologist at the other end of the phone. That practice was one floor above the ER, and I was to report there at 8:00 the next morning.

They had tried one drug—my soon-to-be nemesis, Metoprolol—while I was there, and sent me home with another pill to take a couple hours later that night. I think I had confidence I would "feel better in the morning," and that no further follow-up would be necessary. Ha!

It's funny—even though I was in the ER for only three or four hours, and they did not do anything invasive or extensive, I was flat-out exhausted. Fatigue aside, we did our best to figure it out ourselves. I was curious, of course, and wanted to do anything I could to prevent this only-once-in-a-(my)-lifetime-occurrence. And my wife is a world-class analyst (not to be confused with a finger-pointer or fussbudget). Henceforth, our armchair assessment began.

The next day's initial consultation with the cardiologist was tremendously valuable—even despite my best efforts at self-diagnosis. He spent a great deal of time with us; drawing pictures, loading me down with literature and even offering me his personal cell. number (I hope he doesn't lose his license if the powers that be read this), with a pledge to answer any questions I may have, as he understood the inefficiencies of calling the practice or the hospital. He explained that Atrial Fibrillation is very common—although generally in folks with decades' more tocks on the ticker than me. It is often without a specific or direct cause, and is generally treated very effectively with medication. He was optimistic that I would "convert" soon (was he practicing medicine, or religion?), and that this was a hopeful isolated incident. Now, several skepticism-filled years later, I think he sugar-coated it for me…and in hindsight, I actually appreciate that.

He was consultative and patient, and not arrogantly dismissive of our neophytes' analysis or our Biology 101 discussion questions. Nor our concern that my arrhythmia was self-inflicted by overloading on coffee.

———

FLASHBACK: Finland, the land of coffee and cake…and coffee and coffee and coffee!

I had just returned from a month-long cultural exchange trip with Rotary International. Its purpose was nebulous—simply a "cultural exchange." One of Rotary's themes is Peace Through Understanding, and I know this small trip had a significant impact upon several lives as we grew to know another culture.

I led a group of four young professionals from our district in eastern Kansas. Their application and interview process was exhaustive, as well it should be—in addition to sharing our Kansas culture across the Scandinavian tundra, the five of us were to be in close quarters for a month.

I was glad for the exhaustive process on the front end. This trip was a personal reach for me. I was in my late-thirties, fairly well-ingrained in what I like (and do not like), and in daily personal and professional routines. I was about to be not in control of my schedule for a month. Add in the significant factor that I am by nature an introvert, and I was truly to be out of my comfort zone.

But I applied for the team leader position because I had really enjoyed every Rotary experience I'd had to that date—if I was going to push myself, this was going to be a fascinating way to do it.

We compiled a great team. More significantly, a diverse team. Diverse, anyway, for Kansas. None of them were clones of me 15 years removed, thank goodness. And that was part of what was going to push me—I had to become flexible (yes, dear—me, flexible) to lead them, to allow myself to function in a new and uncontrolled paradigm, and to work together to survive in a foreign country.

"Survive" turned out to not be the right word. We were treated exceptionally well. All our hosts were thoughtful, considerate and warm. But again—every day was a different experience.

As we prepared for the trip over the several months prior to departure, our group gelled. We practiced Finnish vocabulary, figured out technical and personal logistics, divided up personal and group duties, designed our collateral materials and created a presentation on civic, professional, cultural, business and charitable aspects of life as we knew it in America's Midwest. Over the 30 days in-country, we probably made the presentation more than 45 times together as we visited businesses, city halls, and of course, local Rotary clubs.

We all also did that presentation individually for our hosts and their families. Often immediately upon arriving at a new host, and therefore at the end of a long, full day. We were universally exhausted—even the young ones, to say nothing of yours truly. I don't sleep a lot, but I do prefer some quiet down time, especially after long days spread across clumsily-bilingual small talk, intense personal and group conversations, travel across the small but rural district in southwest Finland on the Ostrobothnian coast, new experiences at every turn...and struggling with the language. Despite our best attempts at preparation, every little bit of Finnish that I had managed to cram into my hard head immediately turned to mush as we boarded the Finnair flight in New York. The lovely flight attendants greeted us in Finnish, and they may have been announcing our trip to Mars for all I knew. It was almost scary. Fortunately, the younger and more agile minds in my group had practiced—or retained, anyway—more than I had.

As a whole, the experience was wonderful and reinforced my dedication to a group that had meant, and has come to mean a great deal more to me personally. Rotary is fun for me—a chance to have non-business conversations and fellowship once a week, but also within a remarkable international organization that affords us the infrastructure to do good in every corner of the globe.

But why, you ask, am I boring you with this? Because the timing may be uncanny.

While no medical professional has ever lent any credence to the connecting of the dots, I firmly believe that gallons and gallons of coffee may have been a cumulative trigger (if I lived in California, I could probably sue someone, but I digress...) to my arrhythmias.

I am thankful of the timing for two reasons. First, that my symptoms did not manifest themselves while overseas, and two, that they did manifest themselves less than a fortnight after returning home to Suburbia, Kansas.

While our daily schedules were packed with travel, presentations, and getting to know our local hosts and their families, the one constant was that all revolved around a beverage that has been a strong player in my life.

The Finns truly love their coffee. And by example, they consume more per capita than any other country in the world. Ironically, they also consume more spirits than anyone else in the world (perhaps owing to long, long dark winter months), but that was not a part of my experience. Perhaps to paraphrase President Trump: "Imagine what a mess I'd really be if I were to drink!"

Our days always began with breakfast—often with Finnish staples like salmon, potatoes, breads spread with the super-Vitamin C jam of Sea-Buckthorn berries, reindeer meat and "hirven"—moose! On hurried days perhaps just juice and milk...but always, always our days began and ended with coffee. Always.

I love coffee, the Finns really love coffee, and it is a standard show of hospitality to serve it. Not only with a meal, but at any time that called for a deep conversation, a casual conversation, or just sitting down for five minutes. It is a grievous insult to not accept a cup. And even more so to refuse a refill. They are wonderful hosts, and borderline aggressive in topping off a steaming mug.

I was in heaven. Morning, noon and night...and at every point in between. A conservative estimate is more than a dozen cups throughout the day. Every day. At that point in my life, I was an all-day-long coffee drinker, and it was thrilling to have it presented to me at every turn. No trips to the local shop were necessary—every sit-down at a business or civic or Rotary meeting began with coffee. Oh yeah—cake and other treats usually accompanied the elixir. And it was also rude to attempt to refuse those offerings.

One team member even made a trip through the Finnish medical system, owing to stomach problems that were obviously spurred by the daily overdosing. He was trying to cut down to one cup at each stop, and would eagerly jump at a broadened offering of the national soft drink—an orange soft drink that required an acquired taste. Jaffa had as big a foreign fan as I was of the proletariat coffee. Yum. Yum for all of us.

So yes, by my layman's eye, 30 days of coffee and cake was a clear smoking gun. And yet not one physician in Kansas really even listened to Heather and me try to make this connection. I still wonder....

———

I think my cardiologist made us both feel better. I know I felt better. Especially with the reassurance that my literal (see: sauna/ice-swimming) Finnish immersion had not triggered my latent lame heart. The medical strategy was to not rush into anything. We looked at my calendar (another offense of modern medical practice?), and decided to let the drugs work for a week. I was young, relatively strong, and in decent shape. If I had not converted to sinus (regular) rhythm within that week, we would schedule me for an Electrical Cardioversion.

As thankful as I was for modern American medical expertise, I was doubly grateful for the timing of my incident. What if I had been afflicted with "Bingo Balls" in the Finnish countryside? I had enough trouble not speaking the language—how would I even describe the new and nebulous symptoms, let alone go about getting treatment? And a more probable retrospective concern—would I even have sought professional help? More likely I'd tough it out and wait for the friendly confines of Kansas. Even though I had never personally slogged the morass of our medical-industrial complex, I am fairly certain that my native language and a valid insurance card would be effective step-one tools.

Again, the doctor was very comforting, but as the days dragged on without conversion, The Big Zap began to loom large in my head. I knew in my soul that I was in fine hands and that it was an everyday procedure, but it still felt like a big deal—*because it was happening to ME!*

By now I've had more than a dozen Cardioversions, but I still don't like talking about all of the specifics. The long and the short of it is that they stop one's heart, and then re-start it, hopefully in sinus rhythm. They do put you to sleep to do it, and then electricity is used for the restart.

It's generally performed in the "Cath (catheter) Lab," and really only takes a few hours. For the patient's purposes, it's an all-day deal though. There may be some reason relating to the heart's burden, but I think it's almost entirely the fact that you've been anaesthetized.

Of course you don't want to eat for twelve hours (at least) prior, but I never had any problem on the back end. That is noteworthy because the anesthetics sometimes do not treat me well. It's good in this case because my first Cardioversion was of the Trans-Esophageal Echocardiogram variety. Because of the incumbent esophageal intrusion, one can often have throat irritation...and its best remedy is ice cream on the way home. Who doesn't have a jealous memory of the grade school classmate who recounted meals and meals of ice cream after the exotic-sounding "tonsillectomy?" I needed to fill that childhood void.

My Nantucket Sleighride

THE TRANS-ESOPHOGEAL Echocardiogram part of a TEE-Cardioversion allows a better view of the insides, from the inside.

My TEE allowed them to notice a small hole in my heart. It was congenital, and is not entirely uncommon. We all start out with these small holes, but they grow closed, either in the womb or shortly thereafter. Occasionally, they do not close as they're supposed to. That's mine: an Atrial Septal Defect. Or, as I reflect, its discovery was the beginning of my Nantucket Sleighride....

I do remember the post-procedure conversation with the doctors, but think I was still a little groggy. I could tell, however, that I was in sinus rhythm, and I was thrilled. My now-concluded arrhythmic chapter had only been for about a week, but it felt amazing to have a smooth-firing V6 powering me instead of a rumbly flat-four with one faulty spark plug.

My reaction to the ASD discovery was fairly nonplussed, either from diminished cognitive ability at the moment, or because of the doctors' calm nature. Again, clearly not life threatening—they're getting ready to send me home! But it was certainly enough—for the coming days, weeks, months, and years—to make a guy think about it. In the middle of the workday, driving down the freeway, while nervously exercising, or in the middle of the night.

Sonofabitch. She was right! My fourth-grade teacher, after I had tried out for the lead in the elementary school musical. I thought I was in great shape, because I actually did memorize all the words for the tryout. But the words were the easy part. "Adam, we're going to go in a different direction for you. I can't have you sing. ***You have no rhythm****."*

So, thanks to the "this really is fairly common" medical stance, my discharge was pleasantly efficient. We caught our collective breath (me more than Heather), and drove away smoothly…and straight to the nearest place for a great cheeseburger and milkshake! I needed the nourishment, and ice cream is always a strong palliative.

I remember eating my feast at the kitchen table, and not feeling nearly as bad as I had expected to. I know damn sure I didn't want to admit that, though, and waste any good sympathy. I did agree to take a nap after my late lunch/early dinner.

———

Undressing brought about another surprise and a watchword to potential customers: skin care and preparatory shaving is critical! When I went in to the ER at the initial diagnosis, the EKG leads and IV tape-job were certainly uncomfortable, but I did not think to do anything about them. The small sections of chest and arm hair were not significantly affected. A cardioversion, though, requires clean contact on vast swaths of real estate, front and back.

I had never given any thought to chest hair. My wife likes mine, which is great, and I guess I was cognizant of silver hairs sprouting. In my early thirties I considered this a good sign—silver or grey thickly on top of my head was a wonderful prospect compared to the wiry and thin description that ascribed my dad and his brothers. I clung to the “skip-a-generation” school of layman’s genetics, and hoped I’d have a rich, wavy and distinguished silver mane like my dad’s dad had (and, like my mom’s dad also had).

So…not being a bodybuilder, nor at the beach everyday here in landlocked-land, it never meant much to me. Until I looked at the huge rectangular patch of red naked skin in the middle of my chest. It was tougher to see on my back, as it didn’t stand out like Stan Herd’s first attempt at crop field art. It looked like someone had pressed a steam iron to my chest. Without the sleek pointy end, but it was a big, maybe four-by-eight-inch rectangle smack in the middle of my chest. And the skin was irritated—like that iron had been cranked up to eleven.

I know Heather had seen it while I was knocked out, and probably in preparation too, but I quickly slathered some lotion on the bald spot, covered myself in a shirt, and collapsed into bed. It was a beautiful, clear spring afternoon, and I was going to sleep like an old man. I slept hard, and woke up three or four hours later, ate another snack (with ice cream), and went back to bed.

The next morning I woke up okay and went to work. Still moving gingerly, but I functioned throughout the day. I think some of my timidity was from the skin irritation, some was from general fatigue, and some was from the literal shock to my system. A lot, I'm, sure had to do with the general feelings of curiosity, worry, but mitigated by the palpable relief at having been "fixed."

The next weekend, when Heather was running some errands (and couldn't witness or heckle the disappointing spectacle), I took an electric razor to my torso and evened things out. That's not easy to do, and the remaining hair looked ragged, at best, and the skin looked both fresh and ugly at the same time. On Sunday I learned another lesson—body hair is a great chafing-prevention device. After my morning run, I found further skin irritation…which, in the grand scheme of things, is not a steep price to pay.

Overall, I felt a thousand percent better than I had for the previous week. I know I made a quick mental inventory and leap forward: I feel good, I have a ton of work to do, and the doctors aren't worried—I can put that niggling little ASD out of my head, and get back to normal life. We'll get that fixed at a convenient time…*if it even needs to be repaired,* and a couple days in, I was wholly convinced I was—and would be—fine. I had made it nearly four decades like this—there's no real need to improve upon it. It was nice that the arrhythmia showed up to show the defect to us, but I wouldn't need to revisit that for another four decades. Right? Right. Yeah, right….

Cardioversion, the layman's description:

Most physicians are inherently good communicators, and I believe most of those even refine and improve that skill during their many years of studying, training and practice. For the first week or so of my new-found immersion into being a cardiac patient, my doctor was tremendously patient, educational, and, I now know, full of euphemisms and well-chosen words. I don't mean that caustically—his soft-pedaling of information to me was exactly what I needed.

Atrial Fibrillation *is a "very common, minor irregular rhythm, often easily treated."* Cardioversion *is a "simple procedure where a slight electrical charge is used to get the heart back into its normal, natural rhythm." An* Atrial Septal Defect *is a very small hole in the wall between the upper chambers of your heart. We all start with these holes, and as the heart develops, they generally close. Not always. We'll keep an eye on it, and can easily close it, if necessary."*

No problem, no big deal—I'm young, strong, healthy—these "minor," and "simple" things are not significant setbacks. I trust this smart man to fix it, easily and quickly, and I'll never have to see him again in my life. Especially as this impending little "cardioversion" procedure was to set me straight.

An Electrical Cardioversion is a straightforward procedure. Probably the toughest part of my first one was the simple unknown, especially as the professional and efficient techs prepared all the machinery and the patient.

Most of my cardioversions were elective, or non-emergency procedures. There were a couple times that I was hurried into one, but that was when I was most symptomatic. And those quick ones occurred because it was safer to get me back into rhythm than to continue arrhythmically. Being on a blood thinner is necessary, either on daily doses prior, or they can load you up immediately prior to your procedure. Having been on blood thinners almost throughout since my first episode, I was generally okay to be plugged in.

To do it, they prep and shave the patient. An IV line is started ("Which arm would you like it in, sir?" "Someone else's."), and an EKG is generally run throughout (thank goodness, as I've had more than one cardioversion called off because my body corrected itself at the last minute, and the monitor proves it), and then they're ready. The recently-anesthetized patient never sees them, either before or after, but large conductive paddles are placed on the center of the patient's chest and back. The current runs for less than a second, and generally the heart restarts in-rhythm. Sometimes the first one does not take, and the procedure is repeated...but with higher measures of electricity.

Cardioversions involve a Trans-Esophageal Echo (TEE), which is an imaging procedure. I had had the impression that it was important for them to see my heart in its best detail before flipping the switch, but I now understand it is less concern for the heart's structure, and more to monitor for the presence of blood clots. Good to be cautious, as clots are a significant concern with any type of arrhythmia. And when the heart is restarted using a jolt of electricity, clots can conceivably be jarred loose, sending them northward to bad places.

Three good points about the TEE part of a cardioversion: 1) the monitoring and avoidance of potentially fatal blood clots, 2) they discovered my ASD this way, and 3) it's a terrific excuse for ice cream afterwards.

In my experience, cardioversion works fine, and is relatively painless and easy. I don't, however, want to meet the forward-thinking masochist who created the procedure.

Six Smooth Months

I HAD TWO follow-ups with my regular (soon to be *very* regular) cardiologist, and at each visit he was reassuring and educational. And the communication went both ways—as he educated me to the evils of caffeine, I reassured him that I had cut every drop out of my diet.

I made it through the summer in pretty good shape. No incidents of arrhythmia, so I guess that's better than just "pretty good." We probably began to feel overconfident. And maybe a little cheap. Heather had had a small surgical procedure that September, and all went fine. We had maxed out our significant family insurance deductible for the year, though, and I began to consider making the system work for us for a change.

My frugality was only a portion of it, though. In my then-career I was to get exponentially busier each month

January-June. Therefore, April or May was a particularly awful time for me to have a surgical procedure. Even for what I now know is a fairly small and simple catheter-driven procedure.

So yes, we got cocky and accelerated things. And at the risk of foreshadowing, I in no way hold my cardiologist responsible for my subsequent years of struggle.

"Warn" is not the right word, but he did make me aware of potential future "electrical" problems growing and being exacerbated by any poking and prodding around within the heart. He also made clear the potential difficulties in ablating future arrhythmias once the ASD closure device was in place.

But we did take all necessary steps and waited appropriate amounts of time between steps before leaping into that void. I had a full examination in the late fall. I wore a 30-day event monitor through the month of November. I ramped up on a blood thinner. The event monitor report came back free and clear. We scheduled the procedure to close my defect on December 18.

———

Piece of cake, despite (or maybe because of?) a late pinch-hitter at the plate. The previously scheduled doctor was suffering from the flu. They told me while I was being prepped. Did I mind of they used a sub? If okay to proceed, he'd come by and introduce himself, answer any questions, and we'd forge ahead.

What did I know? What did I care? I had never even met the originally scheduled guy. He had simply been described as "the guy in the practice that does this." Um, okay. Yes, early in the process I was tremendously naïve.

Naïve or not, there was no reason for worry with this, nor frankly, any doctor. Actually, I'll clarify that a little. The first guy was a proud graduate of the school which is the sworn, blood enemy of Heather's alma mater. She was dubious, and that made me have to defend the guy (sight unseen), just for my own peace of mind!

Nonetheless, the scab, who happened to be the head of the practice, was pleasant and gregarious in our hallway consultation, and Heather really enjoyed his pre-game strategy. That right there made me feel good, in my partially-prepped and immobile position.

Back to my description of its resolution—yes, piece of cake. I don't remember much of the goings-on before or after. Part of that is because of my naiveté—when everything is totally unfamiliar, it is tough to internalize much. Especially in times of stress.

I'll qualify that statement a little bit. I was not "stressed" about the procedure—it was routine-ish, I was in otherwise good health and strength, and I was in great hands. I had nothing about which to worry.

The stress was kind of cumulative. The other side of that coin is that I was to be finished! I was thankful that the arrhythmia had allowed us to notice the ASD. I was thankful that I had been well-monitored for eight months, and that this team of professionals thought completely that this was the right strategy for me, and at the right time.

Cool. I had a little incident half a year ago, they watched it, and allowed me to get to this point. Whereby I would soon be better-than-ever, and I could not wait. I figured I'd have an annual checkup for a few years, and then as everything progressed like a normal, healthy person my age should, I'd be off the hook.

And I was especially looking forward to being stronger than I had ever even had potential to be. As my nearly four-decade heart had never worked at 100%, I was going to be in fat city once I was repaired! Any concerns I had internally were usurped by daydreams of Herculean daily energy, increased mental capacity and a springboard into my second trimester of life (and apparently, some blind over-optimism).

More than one joke was made in anticipation of my being bionic. In fact, I proudly borrowed that from my dad, who had had a simple pacemaker implanted about 20 years earlier.

Bionic, strong, better-than-brand-new here I come! I was glad to be there, and I pledged to stay out of there (the hospital) moving forward. I would follow doctors' orders to rehab, and then once cleared, I would even further improve my lifestyle to avoid them molesting me any further.

———

The worst part of that recovery stemmed from my desire to follow orders, down to the syllable for my first 12 hours. With no surgical context in my life, I was scared. And that fear was reinforced because my blood did not clot readily. Nor should it have. For any procedure, they load you up on blood thinners. Especially for cardiac, catheter procedures. When I was in recovery, my heart was pumping and my blood was flowing…right out the small holes in my "leg." Pressure and time are the best ways to staunch blood flow, and I give a gold medal to the 90-pound sprite of a nurse who spent what felt like hours perched on my groin urging me to coagulate.

When I finally did, and that poor nurse was sent to the showers, I was deathly afraid of starting to bleed again. I was told to get some sleep…but to not move. I adhered to the latter, and had no hope at the former. Not only did I not move a muscle, I kept myself rigid and unbending, all night long. I did not sleep. At some point in the wee small hours a new nurse tried to counsel me on relaxation and sleep, but I was a lost cause. I made myself miserable all night, practicing my planking in solitude, but by God, I did not let those tiny wounds open up again! I was sore, head to toe, for several days afterwards.

The overall recovery was simple and quick. I think my mental rehab was the toughest (yes, even from this miniscule procedure). It took me several days to even look at, let alone actively wash the catheter insert points (there were two or three closely-bunched holes at the top corner of my thigh). Mind you, I am meticulous…but

I'm also very queasy. So, I relied upon the tried and true male method of personal hygiene. Soap suds can be made at high points, and then we would be foolish to not use the simple advantage of gravity and pressurized warm water for those suds to flow down and "clean" everything downstream. No problem.

After a few days, once I could bend and flex and move my arms and torso, I again evened out my chest and other shave jobs, and began getting back to normal. Exercise was a slow progression of walking one mile, two miles, three miles, and then mixing in a little bit of light jogging throughout. In less than a month I was fully cleared to begin pursuing better fitness at my own accord.

But little did I know, I would be back sooner than I had expected.

A New Animal

TWENTY-TWO DAYS later, to be exact. I was in Atrial Fibrillation, and it was persistent. They watched me for a little while, but were duly concerned. Concerned enough to zap me. Twice. The first was a wimpy 70 joules, and when that didn't work, they cranked me up to 200. Zappedy-doo-dah, I was back to normal!

Pretty good again. I felt alright, better each day, and was working on getting back into shape. Maybe slowly, but diligently—absolutely every day.

———

And then something again felt a little funny. Not Atrial Fibrillation, but something different. About a week before I was to take a combined business and family trip, I thought I could feel my implanted closure device.

I was deathly afraid it was not seated properly, or I had dislodged it somehow. It may very well have been in my head (the feeling, not the device), but I felt something, and communicated it, earnestly.

My very-responsive cardiologist indulged my neurosis, and pulled me in for a few tests. We started with the ubiquitous EKG, and then I had to come back in the afternoon for a stress test.

I remember feeling a little proud that I was able to keep pushing the stress test. I felt okay, and finally the nurse said I had done more than enough.

The results showed nothing of worry. This was February 7.

———

On February 8th I flew to Sarasota, Florida, for a few days with my dad before we drove across the state for a business meeting. Navigating the airports and the cattle car in the sky was no problem.

I was even maybe a little eager to be stopped by the TSA. The doctors had told me my nickel and titanium device could not be detected, but I had my certificate of ownership at the ready in my wallet. I thought it would be fun to describe to the arbiter of all human safety that I was now mildly bionic. I clearly needed to get out more. And that's part of why I was excited to travel.

The travel was fine, and I made it to town in time for a great fish dinner.

And in the morning I was thrilled to go for a run, along the harbor, in beautiful warm weather. It was great. A grouper sandwich for lunch, a round of golf, and then of course fish again that night.

It all came to a screeching halt the next day, a Saturday. I woke up very early, in a state of Fibrillation. I spent several hours worrying, hoping I would convert, and waiting before telling anyone.

My dad was sleeping late, as he's allowed to do—he's retired! I didn't want to wake Heather with the news, because there was nothing she could do about it—other than worry—and I didn't want to impose that upon her.

I was also biding my time before contacting my primary cardiologist at home. Again, he was great to give me his cell. number, and I did not want to abuse it. So, I waited until 10:00 Eastern time. It was a long, irregular wait for yours truly. This episode seemed more symptomatic than the most recent (which was more symptomatic than its previous, and so on and so on…). I now know the simple answer; it is a progressive disease.

The kindly doctor told me to double up on my Metoprolol, and wait two hours. If I hadn't converted, I should call him back. Yellow Pages open, we began trying to decide between Urgent Cares and a local hospital at about 1:00 pm. *Another lesson to all: when traveling, carry more than a few days' worth of additional medications. Duh.*

One initial phone call indicated that the local Urgent Care would be my most efficient bet. I'm not sure why we thought that. I paid my copay, waited a while, and they told me to go to the hospital. Maybe I should have had Obamacare…?

That sent me walking in, again, to an ER. And this one was a different story than Johnson County, Kansas.

It was noisy and crowded. And by then I had been up more than nine hours. And I hadn't eaten a thing. That, I recall had been a conscious decision. Not a good one, but I remember my thought process. I initially skipped breakfast because I didn't want to eat anything that would exacerbate the arrhythmia. No coffee, for sure. Beyond that, though, I had worried that sugar from fruit, or carbs and sugar from a bagel or a donut, or even toast would be a complicating factor. And by decision-time, I just wanted to get on the road and get this fixed.

So, I was not in good shape at this stroll-in. Add to that the markedly non-serene situation in the ER, and things got worse. As they were attempting to take blood/hook up an IV, I passed out. I might have thrown up, but I'm not sure. We all know I don't like needles, and this was a bad one. I do remember my last sight of that tech. He was digging in my left arm, just like he was trying to ring up a 3:00 am Jamaican Beef Patty at the 7-11 (where he looked more suited to be working, frankly), and then boom. That was the last I saw of him.

I woke up on a hospital bed, perforated and fully plugged in.

By then Heather and my dad had been on the phone all afternoon. With each other, and with my doctor (sorry, Doc—I'll make it up to you).

There was nothing they could do for me at Sarasota Memorial, so they wrote me a prescription for a $150 blood thinner, and sent me on my way. By then it was nighttime. I was exhausted, and of course hungry. We had a grouper sandwich at a wonderful neighborhood dive bar, and went back to my dad's place and crashed.

I flew home the next morning and then went to my local hospital for another Cardioversion on February 11.

Nice vacation. For a "disease" that is not life-threatening, it sure is lifestyle-impinging.

———

The best $30.00 I ever spent, and the worst airline flight I ever took:

When I had my remote incident in Florida, I was eager just to get home.

I felt awful, I hadn't slept much in about 30 hours, and was exhausted. I'd been through a lot: early morning waking with arrhythmia, six hours at least of worry and wait and phone calls with my home cardiologist, time selecting the appropriate venue to treat me (hospital, hospital ER, cardiology practice, or urgent care), time to get there and hobble in, waiting and going through the co-pay and registration and initial consultation at an urgent care, travel to the hospital ER, surviving an *aggressive yet untalented needle-poker, surviving passing out from that IV attempt and allowing another, waking up prostrate in a hospital room, waiting for hours for a consultation and direction, finally being dismissed, finding a pharmacy to fill my $150 prescription, finally making it to a light dinner of a fish sandwich and iceberg lettuce salad in a plastic boat (which tasted great!), and then sleeping a little bit before fighting my way to the airport the next day.*

Whew. Thankfully, Heather had helped change my plane ticket. I didn't need to wrangle with that, but I had to wrestle myself through spring breakers and nonagenarians to get to my airplane.

I was not ashamed to take some of the best advice I've ever had—I took a wheelchair through the airport. When first suggested to me, I immediately dismissed it—those are for sick people (and nonagenarians). But as I realized how worn out I was, I quickly warmed to the idea.

Curbside check-in is a great convenience. It's even better when you can request a wheelchair from your skycap. I did so with a ten-dollar-bill. He initially protested, as providing wheelchair service is just part of the job, but I was hoping he would find me his best buddy in the building to be my escort. He took my money and scampered off to find the right guy.

Almost immediately he was back, with that best buddy and a shiny old wheelchair in tow. I was thrilled to see him, and I began offering "I feel bad...I'm not really sick..." but I was frankly, exhausted, and just concluded with "Thank you...and my doctor thanks you. I'm glad to be able to get home for emergency surgery tomorrow."

I might have stretched that a little, but not by much—they did have me slated for a Cardioversion the next morning. Not totally an emergency, but not scheduled ahead of time either. But it would give me some much-needed relief. And I was almost there.

My man wheeled me smoothly and quickly through the main lobby. He slowed a little as we approached the security slalom. But only a little. He cajoled himself past the outer edge of the line, and proudly pushed my right up to the front. I did my best to look sickly as he handled my carryon and I stepped out of the chair to be inspected and pass through the checkpoint. I was almost home.

We had a leisurely roll down the concourse to my gate where he helped me stake out a seat. He offered to stay with me, but I knew that was superfluous, and not a good use of his time. I'm happy to be a good tipper, but I didn't want to be responsible for forty minutes of his idle time. Besides, there were real sick people who could use this chair!

Before he departed, we checked in with the gate attendant. Fully complemented with shiny wheels, I asked to be in the pre-board group. Sure, no problem.

So we got me staged for the little wait, and I sat quietly with my briefcase on my lap, as I gauged traffic before the cattle-call lineup. A couple of sawbucks reinforced my appreciation for my savior, and he did move on, eager to be of real help in a building in dire need of it.

And then the circus came to town. Or rather, the Aquarium came to my gate, on its way to my city.

I had been looking forward to a nice, quiet nonstop flight home. I was confident in a seat up front, and I would be safely allowed easy ingress and egress. And then my lovely wife would pick me up at the airport (and probably with a bottle of cold water and a Dairy Queen Blizzard to comfort me).

Nothing doing. I was on a celebrity flight. At first there were probably a half-dozen advance men and handlers. They created a little buzz in our corner of the concourse, and passengers everywhere were self-inducing whiplash looking for the celebrity causing the commotion. As the handlers cleared the way for an electric cart to plow through the middle of the concourse, the mystery deepened. The cart carried a large plastic crate. And upon its arrival at my (yes, MY) gate, right about at my feet, three of the guys wrestled it off the cart and up near the gate's door to the jetway.

We were bewildered, but the buzz was growing. Finally, after fifteen minutes of people milling about and stepping on my front-row feet, a giddy stewardess announced our celebrity passenger. A sea turtle. Yep.

A damned sea turtle that its entourage seemed to have confused with the second coming of Christ.

I had a headache, I ached everywhere, come to think of it—I had spent eight hours in a hospital, eaten very little and slept even less, and so I was justifiably cranky. I did not want to share my airliner with a turtle in a box.

———

They called for boarding. I, the sick people and the nonagenarians had to wait to get on the plane until the damned turtle and her team of world-savers had taken over the first two rows of the airplane.

Fine...I can live with being in Row Three. Just don't bother me. Let me read my book or nap in peace.

Nothing doing. Gertrude's handlers were justifiably proud of their charge, and they were eager to evangelize her charming presence. Being at the front of the plane, they were able to do so to each and every passenger boarding. The flight did not leave on time.

———

I'm a tall person, and as such always seek an aisle seat. It's slightly easier on my back and knees to be able to stretch into the walkway on occasion. It is also a higher-traffic location. I endured three hours of looky-loos hitting me on the head as they grasped for my seatback on their wobbly way to have a word with the damned turtle...or better yet, one of her vociferous now-celebrities-themselves handlers.

I had twenty minutes of relief when the captain, sounding nearly as giddy as the nitwit gate attendant, announced that they were going to be able to take Gertrude out of her box and show her off throughout the plane. Oh, goody.

On the bright side, they leapfrogged my row and began abusing the aisle passengers in every row behind me as they muscled the turtle down the plane and back.

While I was at the gate, and while sitting on the plane waiting for the circus to be seated, I told Heather that I was flying with a turtle (I didn't know they could fly?).

She did not make the full connection, though, until she waited for me at the airport and television crews began setting up for "the shot."

And of course, the turtle and crew deplaned before me, the real sick people, and the nonagenarians. And then they stopped right there. I had hoped they might be in a hurry to get her into some real water, but her time was better served sharing her turtle message to all of Kansas City...right at the bottleneck point in the gate area.

It's a nice story, isn't it? It's my genuine pleasure to be able to share it....

Gee, does AFib make an otherwise-amiable guy grumpy? Ugh.

A New Fluttering Friend

THE NEXT MONTH I drove myself back to the hospital. This time in a non-emergency situation. I was going in for a sleep study. There is an apparent and very real link between Sleep Apnea and Atrial Fibrillation. Let's check it out.

It was a bitter cold Sunday night. We had a normal dinner, albeit several hours earlier than usual. I had to check myself in at 8:00 pm. While arrhythmia does make a guy fatigued, I do not go to bed quite that early. It took at least two hours to get all hooked up anyway. This was significantly more invasive than a simple heart monitor. In addition to the torso and arm torture I had anticipated, I also had a half-dozen leads stuck to my head. My head! In my hair. Great gobs of contact-improving jelly. Gross.

When fully attached, the nurse asked me what I thought was an incongruous question: did I use sleeping pills? And if not, would I like one anyway?

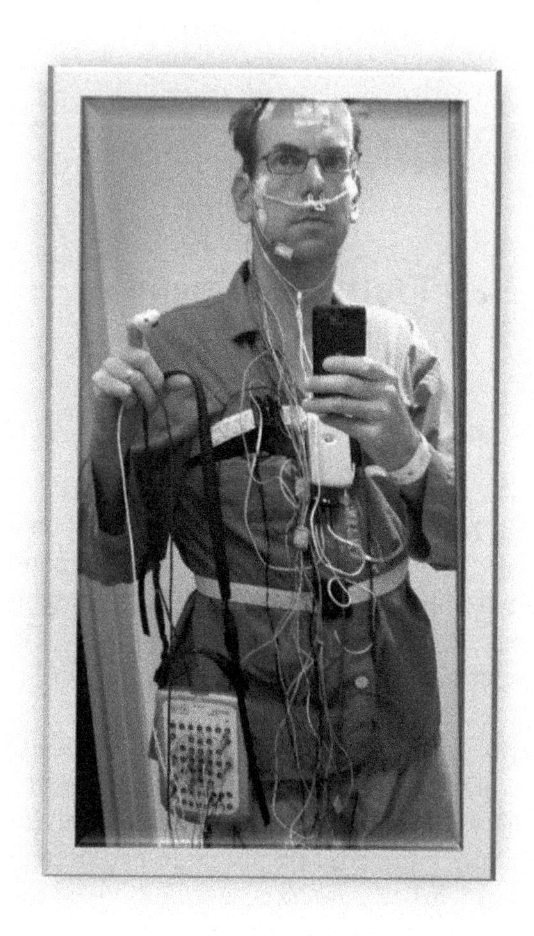

Um, no, I don't. And wouldn't that invalidate the sleep study findings anyway, if I'm knocked out cold? I didn't think that would be an accurate gauge of my normal sleeping patterns.

The nurse was perfectly nice, but I got the distinct impression I was the first person to ever push back on this question. As she described her medical perspective, I bought in, partially.

Strangely, folks sometimes had trouble falling asleep while in the hospital (um…I could write three chapters on that myself, and did, but then in an unprecedented act of mercy to readers, deleted them)—let alone when one has thousands of contact points leaving more skin covered than exposed. A sleep aid would simply allow me to fall asleep, and then they would actually have a better time tracking my patterns.

Okay—I let her give me half a pill. And I guess it worked. I woke up at my normal time, feeling wholly *un*rested, and then let her unhook me.

In an attempt to maintain normalcy, I raced home, took one shower to un-goop myself, exercised, took another shower, then dressed and made it to the office for a normal Monday morning meeting.

A few days later they called with the results. No sleep apnea. No smoking gun. Back to the drawing board.

———

One month later:

I pushed through a moderate workout on our basement treadmill, came to the kitchen and finished my vitamins with a tall glass of very cold water. And I felt it—my heart was not happy.

In our house, we've got the early mornings and late nights covered. But not together. I love the early morning, and Heather likes to sleep in a little. I pondered and puttered around the house for maybe thirty minutes, debating what to do. Drive right to the hospital myself, ask Heather for a ride (and thereby ruin her day), or go about normal business and let the wonder drugs take over, eventually?

Leaning toward the last option, I made my way upstairs slowly and didn't say anything. I showered, but was then short of breath getting dressed.

Over the course of the now-four-year saga, Heather would often pick up on something being wrong (it could be anything), and invariably ask: "are you in arrhythmia?!?!" It took us a while, but we finally agreed that she could assume, at all times, I was not, and that I would tell her when I was. Even at this point, just six months in, I was leery of worrying her. But I was even more leery of this episode. I asked her to feel my pulse, and in the same breath told her to not worry, because *I was* going to the doctor.

This episode was tougher than previous ones, and that fact helped sway me to take action right away. I'm glad I did. As I walked across the hospital parking lot, severe lightheadedness caused me to crouch down and place my hands on the curb. Of course I didn't want to make a scene, so I was scanning the area in case I needed to ward off any helpful attendants or ambulance drivers.

Having made it inside the building, I took the elevator upstairs, and the cardiology practice quickly swooshed me into an exam room and began the hook-up process.

———

There are a few different types of arrhythmia. My first flavor was fibrillation in the atria, or upper chambers of the heart. Today's form was flutter, also on the second floor.

Both are "electrical" problems, and neither is particularly life threatening. As I was learning, and would well know in years forward, they certainly have the capability to significantly impair one's lifestyle. Not everyone's mind you, as there are millions of Americans who suffer from Atrial Fibrillation asymptomatically. I know "suffer" does not sound like the right word—if they're *asymptomatic,* what difference does it make? Well, while they might not directly feel the aberrant beats, they may be unknowingly fatigued, and simply be used to it. They also are at a severely heightened risk for stroke.

The electrical malfunctions that cause each affliction are markedly different. Fibrillation is totally irregular. My layman's description is that the electrical signals that are supposed to be in charge become completely random; in location, direction, and frequency. The comparison is like the difference between a Direct Current power source, and a springtime lightning storm. No rhyme or reason to it, and certainly no "rhythm" to it. As these incomplete signals trigger poorly-timed beats, the heart's chambers cannot work in synchronicity, and they absolutely do not work at top efficiency or efficacy.

That last sentence still rings true for instances of Atrial Flutter, but the electrical scenario is different from the randomness of Fibrillation. The Flutter signals circulate, literally, like on a horizontal racetrack around the walls of the atria. And *race* is absolutely the best word for it. One's heart rate while in Atrial Flutter can commonly eclipse 200 beats per minute.

I felt like I was hit by a freight train. I could not breathe fully, I could hardly walk across a parking lot, and nearly couldn't see. These symptoms grew over the course of the couple hours I was afflicted. I say that because yes, I did drive myself to the hospital, and felt absolutely dreadful once I stepped out of my car. This was appreciably more chronic than when the symptoms began a little more than an hour earlier. At its outset I did try to forge ahead, and wasn't in bad shape as I climbed the fifteen stairs to our bedroom. While I was showering it got worse. Dressing was even tougher. After mentioning it to my wife, it was all downhill, somewhat thankfully. Descending the stairs was easy. I slipped on some loafers (no shoelace tying, or I would have been in real trouble), and then dropped in to my car.

Twelve minutes after backing out of my garage was when I felt in real trouble. When I took my parking lot breather, I looked back to the car. I knew I had a bottle of water there (I did not think it was cold—nor did I know of any connection to vagally-induced arrhythmia), and I thought one little sip might help me feel better and make it inside to salvation. Either a sip, or pouring it over my head.

I only needed a matter of maybe thirty seconds to catch my breath and resume the trip. And once I was safely inside the second-floor, elevator-accessed office suite, they quickly diagnosed the Flutter. I thought it sounded more benign than the four-syllable affliction, but I sure did not feel more benignly-hit by that freight train.

My heart was running around 200 bpm, and that means that just little whispers of oxygenated blood are moving. At least with Fibrillation, one occasionally gets a full pump. This was tough, and I don't think I even made it home. They pretty quickly made a decision to zap me (perhaps at least partially because I had not eaten anything yet that morning), so they rolled me down the hall to the Cath Lab and Heather altered her schedule and joined me.

Another day shot, and another cheeseburger and milkshake. Pretty tough way for a guy to treat himself to a (rare) greasy lunch.

———

As the Flutter onset was pretty quick and pretty significant, we immediately discussed its fix. An Ablation for Flutter is fairly straightforward. Easy for me to say—I only had to not eat, show up, and have faith.

A Catheter Ablation means that the heart is accessed via a catheter that is run through veins or arteries. It is "easy" to reach the area they need to fix for Flutter, and the proper blood vessels are accessed from the groin. The same route as my implanted closure device of just a few months prior.

———

Sign me up. On March 20, I went downtown for a Flutter Ablation. That all went swimmingly—they were sure they hit the circuits that brought on the Atrial Flutter. Great!

But while they were rooting around in there, they triggered Atrial Fibrillation. Again. I hung around the hospital hoping for "conversion,' and when I again proved stubborn, they zapped me on the morn.

The Catheter Ablation really didn't bother me at the time, and I don't think it bothered the nurses who were very professional. There were two tough parts. The first was (again) trying to get the bleeding to stop after the procedure, and after of course they removed the catheter; I seemed to have been more awake this time. The other tough part for me was bathing for the first several days. And that's only because I'm a baby. Now, three-plus years later, a tiny venous catheter insertion point wouldn't even cause a wince; back then, it was major surgery.

Weary, Fatigued, Clumsy and Frustrated

I THINK EVERYONE in the cardiology practice began to forget my name. I went through the balance of the year and nearly all of the next without incident. Without major incident, anyway.

Through the nearly two years of keeping my hide intact, we did change medications a little bit. Part of that was out of concern for efficacy, and part was because I was miserable.

No medication is foolproof, though, and I was in and out of arrhythmia occasionally.

I learned to live with the situation—mostly with the side effects of the medication. I was more fatigued, on a near-constant basis, than I had ever been in my life, and I was cold. COLD! Always. That was awful. Especially as the heat of a Kansas summer subsided. The fall was actually a little more pleasant, as it provided some relief from our Texas-wannabe air conditioning.

I now know that Metoprolol is one of the drugs that aggravates this effect the most. I know my cardiologist had great reasons for prescribing it, but I was slowly realizing that it would be a problem, long-term. I had never been even moderately bothered by cool or cold temperatures—it might have been my Minnesota roots or especially my Germanic stubbornness—but it was now bothering me on a daily basis.

A much better description comes from a real (literary, not medical) professional. John Irving's character Juan Diego describes "the ennui, the inertia, the sheer sluggishness, he'd so often complained about to (his doctor)." Months later in *Avenue of Mysteries,* another physician "must have known that Juan Diego wasn't acting; his return to torpor, to a diminished level of alertness and physiological activity, was evident to everyone."

Prolol torpor aside, I need to point out one more byproduct of arrhythmias: clumsiness. To be more precise, fatigue exacerbates, or even creates, clumsiness. As the hours wore on during days, and as days wore on during the week, I would be more and more run-down. And when one is physically worn-out, one carries oneself differently. I know I was less alert, less self-aware.

During examinations and even routine checkups, it's commonly asked: "have you blacked out, fallen down, during exercise or the normal course of the day?" Of course this is a major concern for any heart condition, and especially conditions that affect blood flow and efficiency. I had never lost consciousness—largely because I learned to live within my symptoms, grabbing hold of a chair as I rose, making sure to notice the top step, not bending down or straightening up too quickly or frequently.

But they never ask: "have you skinned your knuckles, missed a step but caught yourself, banged into a door, been forced to sit quickly?" I had done all of the above, and more. Most were simple, generally not painful not dangerous. But, like a lot of things down this road, they can be cumulative, and that's when it's most bothersome. A sock drawer to the ankle, a hand slipping from a doorknob, or a repeatedly untied shoe—they all add to the fatigue and the malaise. I never passed out, but I did miss a step once…but it didn't really count as an official missed step, so I did not report it (of course, nothing major ever happened when I was wearing a Holter Monitor or an Event Monitor). We have a living room that is sunken by three steps. I think I changed my mind which direction I was going, and lost track of the ups and downs. In doing so, I "athletically" dropped and rolled somehow, and did not hurt myself. I did stay down for a couple minutes, in an attempt to recover my pride (even without an audience) and swallow my mounting frustration.

Beta Blockers as athletic enhancement?

My favorite cardiologist was appropriately low-key in his description of my new drug at its outset. He described the specific medical effects, and how beta blockers in general were widely and very effectively used to remedy Atrial Fibrillation and a host of similar rhythm maladies.

He even went so far as to mention that they've had widespread use as aids in sports where "slowing down" was a benefit. Great—golf season is upon us! I've consistently had a decent game, but I've never been able to make up serious ground on the green. As he described the "side effects," I pretty much only heard that I was going to be able to putt better. As the body's internal receptors are modulated, physical motions can become smoother. Driving and chipping be damned—I was going to be a machine on the short stuff!

It didn't work. In retrospect, I now know why. 1) I was a pretty standard 18-handicapper. In order to capitalize on the minuscule effect of the drug, I needed to be a real athlete, with the ability to put it close every time. Maybe a single-digit guy sinks one extra putt a week. For me, it did not register. And 2) the other effects of the drugs were a thousand percent more significant. The principal complaints from Metoprolol (and all "prolols," as it turns out) are near-perpetual feelings of coldness--never being able to be warm, and significant fatigue. Combined with the body's already-compromised efficiency at blood-pumping, I was a wreck.

As I consider those dark months of prolol-servitude, I do wish I had been more vocal with my complaints. There are (I now know, much more than I'd like to know) other drugs. They all work differently and with different efficacies...in different people. But, with my neophyte's knowledge or lack thereof, I was primarily concerned with following the doctor's orders exactly. He prescribed this to me for a reason. And he did mention that there were others, but in his opinion, this was the best one for me. It's only logical for this one to work best, and all others to be inherently inferior. I therefore did not push it.

For my own self-preservation of course, I wish I had. For Heather's sake, as well, I really wish I had. Yes, we were managing and alleviating some very real concerns, but the net result was that I was more miserable! I am lucky that my spouse is a wonderful caretaker. And I am glad, for both of us, that a lot of worry was alleviated. But I am certain that she was as tired of hearing about me being cold and tired, tired and cold, as I was of being it.

———

My recollection of the timing is hazy, and there was a lot of forth-and-back through these 20 months. I moved from the hated Metoprolol to Flecainide Acetate. Perhaps more accurately, I "broke through" the Metoprolol, and then broke through the Flecainide.

And that's what got me back in lockup, on November 11. I was not able to take in the wonderful Veterans' Day parade in historic Leavenworth, KS. I was mired in

Johnson County, with tubes and wires upsetting my sensibilities.

———

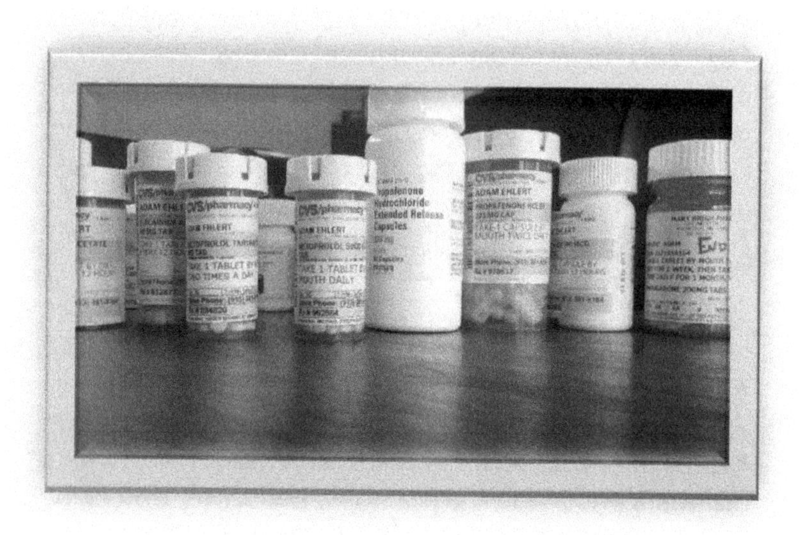

It's also important to note that there many variants within each drug and its family. Adjusting doses is one variable that can be effective once "tuned" right. Adjusting within each family can also work. Metoprolol Tartrate works differently from Metoprolol Succinate ER (commonly abbreviated on the pharmacy label as "Metoprolol Succ," which is precisely my wearied point).

Beyond the Beta-Blockers, Amiodarone works differently from Propafenone, which is different from Diltiazem, also different from Dofetilide, and even good old Flecainide works differently.

I've been on them all (and briefly a few others) at one point or another—and often one in conjunction with another. Despite my reminders for personal vigilance and to be engaged in one's medication, I implore you, from the safety of my armchair—ALWAYS follow your doctors' instructions. Exactly. I've been on what felt like Yahtzee-cup combinations of "rate control" drugs and "rhythm control" drugs. And just as they all work differently; they all interact differently. The prescribing professionals know how—I do not.

My final bit of soapboxing here is to reflect fondly on my time with Flecainide. After the pitfalls of prolols (and especially after I "broke through" their efficacy), Flecainide was my salvation. At least for a little while. I began on moderate doses, just 50 milligrams. As the months wore on, that grew. My prescribed amount was 200 mg. daily, with near carte blanche to use it as my "pill in pocket." You betcha—as symptoms hit, I could pull that sucker out and pop it for near-instantaneous relief...temporary as it was to be.

———

I was having a hard time believing it. It seemed I was out of options. Frustrating. Curious. Infuriating. And yet I couldn't accurately, or fairly, direct my anger at any one particular person or any particular faction of the medical industrial complex.

I was trading calls with cardiologists, and by then, trying to do a little research on my own. In theory, I am dead-set against armchair medicine. Especially layman's armchair medicine.

I think I'm also sensitive to arm's-length medicine. As kind as my first, primary cardiologist was to give me his cell. number, I was cautious of overusing it, and more cautious of putting him in a bad position. I think I did recognize that he could not diagnose over the phone. It would have been unfair for me to hope that he could have a conversation about my all-encompassing situation and history. And it would have been ludicrous to expect him to change my prescriptions over the phone. Ultimately not good medicine for the patient, and just as importantly, I do hold respect for the medical process.

I'm also sensitive to over-consulting a dear childhood friend who now happens to be a cardiologist. By my four-states-removed-perception, he is a tremendous physician. I also know him to be a well-rounded citizen, a great family man, and a whole lot of other things that are diametrically opposed to where we may have been trending in high school.

He has been an absolute salvation, talking me down from trees at times with doses of perspective, and also reinforcing my concerns, and yes, empathizing with my feelings of frustration. Having that sounding board helped keep me somewhat sane, and also helped me navigate the morass.

With that, his ethics are peerless, and I hope to remain a good friend by not asking him to compromise them. I did not ask him to second guess or speak ill of my other physicians. Or diagnose me from afar, or out-prescribe the plan my local doctors were administering.

I mention my "local" doctors here because my pal's perspective was helpful in feeling good about them from the outset.

When the Atrial Fibrillation began, his cautious sagacity reinforced that AFib is common and he was glad I took myself to the hospital. He knew my local hospital, and he also knew several of my local physicians. He had done his residency at the Mayo Clinic, and crossed paths with, or had heard reputations of several of them, including my primary cardiologist. In fact, one almost bought the other's house, as one was transitioning in to Rochester, and the other was on his way out. Small world.

After my first Cardioversion, and the ASD was discovered, he (appropriately) talked me out of doing anything drastic. My dad had had some work done at the Minneapolis Heart Institute, and he has been going to Mayo for an annual physical for decades. My dad was eager to suggest that I go to either of those for further evaluation, treatment, and maybe ultimately for the ASD fix.

My friend assured me that my ASD very likely caused the AFib, and that was great news—to have a smoking cause-and-effect gun. The prescribed local protocol was well-diagnosed, and routine. He was familiar with my physicians, and told me, frankly, that I would not find better elsewhere, and that I was really fortunate to have this resource eleven minutes from my front door.

His personal and unclouded professional opinion was that I would only complicate things for myself by heading to Minnesota. Even going for a second or third opinion would be superfluous and would cloud the issues. Amen.

As my situation dragged on and on, and I was clearly not a one-and-done fix, I was even more thankful that I had a full stable of experts here at home. I cannot attempt to count the number of trips I made to my local team and hospital. The most quantifiable way would be to dig through my credit card statements and tally my $55.00 co-pay charges. I can only imagine how difficult this can be for patients that need to drive an hour or two, or a full day, or get on an airplane to seek consultation.

———

So, come late October, I had a long talk with my pal on a Saturday afternoon. It was a beautiful day, and I was driving home from playing tennis. He knew where I was, physically and mentally. And in his medical opinion, I was approaching a crossroads. We talked for a long time. So much so that I was able to park the car, wander around my front yard enjoying the autumn sun, and make notes on a coffee napkin I pulled from my car's emergency supply.

I thought he was borderline nuts when he mentioned it, and I probably only remember it because I scribbled it down, and then occasionally looked at it for six months while it gathered dust in my garage.

He described two options—surgical and medical. I did not place a lot of water in the surgical bucket. Drugs sound great—even one that requires a three-day lockup to get started! He referred to its technical name, and it took me a little bit to reconcile when my local guy referred to its brand name. Tikosyn—sign me up! The cryptic "Maze Procedure" note would continue its dust-gathering on my garage shelf.

He was cautious in mentioning my wonder drug, primarily I think because of the kidney concerns (that necessitate the three-day stay). He was even more cautious about mentioning the mysterious surgical option. I think he was going to great lengths to practice the "do no harm" doctrine, by not getting me excited about some options that may or may not be the right fit, and therefore causing fits with my local doctors. And I think I realized that—I certainly did not want to go into an appointment with "I heard about this," and "I saw this on Al Gore's Internet." That's not going to result in good medicine for me, it's not good use of my physicians' time, and I would not want the grapevine to finger my friend from another Midwestern city as being a pipeline feeding a know-it-all patient. But it's a fine line between being educated and advocating for oneself. When in doubt, more information is better—especially when gleaned from a trusted advisor.

There was really no option. Cutting was going to be the last (and hopefully unnecessary) option. I was optimistic about Tikosyn. Its efficacy was strong, and its side effects were minimal—provided one makes it through the first five supervised doses.

The Tikosyn condition does beg one question that was never addressed in discussing the other, previous drugs. What is its efficacy, its duration, and the chance of "breaking through" it? Those questions had never crossed my mind to ask. And while I do not think the doctors were necessarily omitting anything, they certainly did not offer any inkling in that direction.

It's entirely possible that I was simply being dense, as I was transitioned from product to product. I continued to take "this one is your best option now" at face value. Duh—I understand, believe, and trust you that this is the best option. Why was it not earlier? Why is this one now? How long can I hope to be on it—or, how long until I can hope to be off it?

That last unsaid question belies an optimism that I held in the deep dark recesses throughout. Again—this is not life "threatening;" it does not totally cripple me; I am forty years old; I am in otherwise really pretty good health. *This cannot last*. It will not be a pervasive issue through the rest of my life. They know what they're doing, and nobody seems overly concerned about it.

It's inevitably going to improve. I will think back, decades from now, at that nice little diversion. It was frustrating at the time, but overall I really can't complain. I have a strong desire to control what I can control, and do my best to stay out of the hospital. I now have the added benefit and peace of mind that I have been inspected every way through Tuesday—the doctors, reams of them, see nothing worrisome. Great! I am in control of my destiny. I'll exercise and eat right--piece of tofu cake. That core value will serve me well in the long, long, long run. This was one small blip on the radar. Right? Right. Yeah...right.

I think my naiveté and inherent optimism led me to complete confidence in my hopeful friend dofetilide. As much as I thought I was a little bit educated as a patient, I still had very little overall context, and of course, zero biological training.

Great—Tikosyn will (now) be the best fit for me. It sure sounds like a wonder drug, and the only reason they've been holding out on me is because of the requisite three-day lockup. Damn insurance boogiemen. While cooling one's heels in the hospital is never fun, at least that's really all I was to be doing. No cutting, no real blood. I could handle that. Especially because my salvation was in sight!

But my salvation did not come overnight. Or over another night. Or another. So yes, once I was fully loaded onto the dofetilide train, I still had not converted yet. Zap, zap again.

This was now nearly two years from my first incident/diagnosis—and I walked out of the hospital with renewed vigor. Yet again. Another Dairy Queen Blizzard, and I was ready to roll.

Devastation; Another Failure

I ROLLED FOR six months. The next spring, I was startled, a little worried, a little close-mouthed, and simultaneously devastated. Capital-D Devastated.

I take my Tikosyn RELIGIOUSLY. Every twelve hours. No more than a 30-minute variation, and even then a variation is as rare as a Travis McGee steak.

I had been singing the drug's praises for these holy six months. It felt like a little secret—they had been holding out on me, and finally allowed me into the secret society. The initiation was a hard-fought four or five days in my local institution of higher boredom and sleep prevention.

I had even been a loyal Tikosynist after three straight months of logic-defying price hikes. No amount of cajoling pharmacists or railing at insurers could reverse it or even make sense of it.

Nonetheless, I brought my blank check each month to the drugstore, and was darn near happy to pay for it. I still had that feeling in my head that this was not to be perpetual, but if it took a year or two to re-train to a natural rhythm, that was worth any price.

And then I felt betrayed. How could this happen? How? Why? What am I doing wrong? This is not right! All my eggs were firmly ensconced in this basket. And the basket was apparently named Hindenburg.

———

Betrayed, desperate, worn-out, figuratively and literally. Frustrated and concerned.

I also felt bad for Heather. I worried about work—this past year was a decent one; what was going to happen when I was further compromised, absent, or simply further down-energy? I worried about friends and family who had been concerned about me. I worried about additional projects I had taken on, and others I hoped to undertake.

After all these years, after all these compromises of time, energy, family and business, it was not supposed to work this way. It was not supposed to drag on.

Dammit—this is a simple problem—why can they not fix it?!?!?

Atrial Fibrillation is for old people. Heart problems are for people who eat fast food every day.

If I'm this tired, cold and frustrated at forty, whatinthhell is fifty and beyond going to feel like? Not right, not fair, and absolutely not fun.

———

Apparently I was not the only one at the end of my rope. My Electrophysiologist's cursory command was: "Go see the surgeon. Here's his number."

Out of options, I dutifully dialed and made an appointment. On the bright side, he fit me in for an appointment in just a couple of days. Surgeons might be eager to cut.

———

Canine Therapy

My morning went out the window. And it was doubly unfortunate because the day was the prettiest weather we'd had so far this year. Pale, high blue sky, with a breeze so light it could also be described as pale.

I didn't sleep much. My heart went out of rhythm around midnight. As the hours ticked by (with regular intervals, unlike myself), I scaled back my plans. I cut out my first weekday morning outside run, reluctantly. I then cut out even a modest walk with the dog. I rolled myself out of bed an hour later than usual, unhappy and unrested. Unable to do anything other than wait an hour for the doctors' office to open. And hope that my drugs would work, and that a call would not be necessary.

No avail, either way. They called me in for a 10:00 EKG. "Yep, you're in AFib, but it looks moderate and controlled." That makes me feel better....

Doc's directive: keep doing what I'm doing. Call when I return to sinus rhythm, or call Friday if I'm still fibbing out and we'll come up with a plan. Oh, and also make an appointment to discuss "cryo-ablation." I remember, we discussed this six months ago, when debating Tikosyn vs. surgery. At the doctor's less-than-overwhelming recommendation, I opted against speaking with the surgeon. But here I am again.

So, feeling a little sorry for myself, I took my time getting home. And then moved slowly when there. Running through scenarios and timing in my wearied head. None good. None fun.

But I'm glad I was taking my time. I decided to take the dog for a walk. We went slow and enjoyed it. At two opportunities we chose the longer route. After the second one we passed a workman and his truck and trailer. It was a beauty; Harley-Davidson paint job, decals, and bullet-hole appliques in the driver's door. The man was standing behind his rickety trailer, peeling an orange and throwing the scraps mostly on the ground near the trailer. I think his aim was off because he was watching Moxie and me.

"What color do they call that?"

"She's fawn, which is only about 6% of Dobermans."

"Wow—she's beautiful. I really miss 'em. I've had four Dobies in my life and they are the greatest. I've got

a black Rottie now—I've never had one before, and I love her to death—but boy, I really miss those Dobies."

"Thank you. She's our first Doberman, and we feel really lucky. She's awesome."

"Aw, I'm happy for you. You enjoy that dog—she'll really take care of you. Have a good day."

And there it is. My day got better.

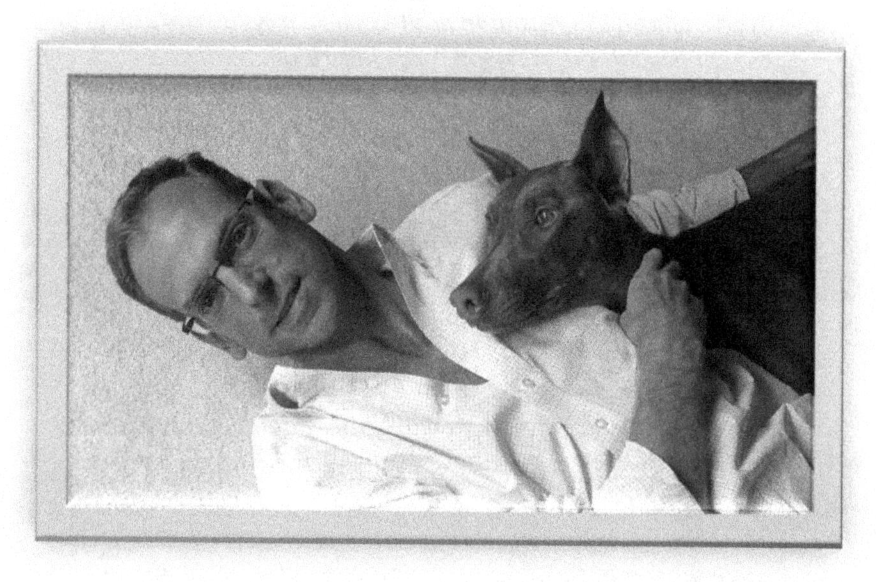

———

As Heather and I tried to take stock of this next chapter, we recalled the less-than-lukewarm medical-speak description of "the surgeon." I believe my EP had, six months ago during the meds vs. surgery debate, described "one guy (in the practice downtown), *who is interested in* this area."

"Not a ringing endorsement" was how this layman interpreted that recommendation six months ago. As I began educating myself in the surgical world, I realized that a medical "interest" is perhaps a field of specialty. Not a passing hobby or sidelight, as I first interpreted the endorsement.

Nevertheless, Heather accompanied me to the consultation, and we were dubious at best upon entering. After following labyrinthine channels to find the office within the under-construction downtown hospital. (And again—how do real sick people do this? It took us, two fully able-bodied, semi-intelligent people—one with a good sense of direction—more than ten minutes to follow the map the kind docents placed in our hands, reconcile that "map" with the disparate signage, and find the right part of the right building, and the right elevator to take us to the right floor. And this was after fifteen minutes in the European-width parking garage. Ugh.).

So we made the appointment, and after not much of a wait we were graced with the presence of the surgeon. We were leery to start, but we quickly warmed to the guy. He was full of gregarious enthusiasm, boundless experience and expertise, and lots of scribbles, drawings, and notes upon the exam-table sanitary paper.

We left with our confidence nearly matching his, and Heather clutched that exam-table paper (butcher's paper?) like it was the Magna Carta. And maybe, hopefully that is an apt analogy. If this scribbled doctrine could make peace between my heart and its environment, then perhaps I could live a free and fulfilling life.

———

There's a fine line between doing one's homework, and overdoing it.

Heather and I both left the initial surgical consultation feeling as strong about the process, procedure, and surgeon as was possible. Good deal, case closed. Any further analysis can only lead in one direction. And yet that's what we did.

In retrospect, of course it was the right move. It's almost never a good idea to accept a first offer, and that's what this felt like, especially in retrospect. In that now-careful consideration, it's particularly clear that it was unclear which procedure was being proffered. I know it was not the open-heart cut-and-sew maze surgery. It was one form of the "Maze," but I'm not sure if it was the Mini, or the Cryo, or some sort of other hybrid.

Part of this confusion was attributable to our naiveté. Part of it directly to near-blind optimism. But the real bulk of the confusion lies at the hands of the provider. He did spend a fair amount of time with us, but he did not discuss the totality of the universe of work in this area, and how in his opinion, his procedure was to be the best for me. His M.O. was clear (now); he had one area of expertise, and he was wholly proficient in performing this one procedure. I was a fish referred to him on a platter, and his place was not to determine how best to fillet me—his job was only to fillet me in the manner he knows. We never even discussed the options—either bigger or smaller.

By simple means of having been referred to him, I had passed all qualifications. I was there, I was otherwise healthy, I had good insurance, and I was at the end of my rope.

Even with the lack of clarity on the overall procedure, I did glean that he had planned to go in through the ribs. Strangely, that makes me cringe. He did clearly state that it was painful, but he then went a long way to state that this is a lot simpler than a fully "open" heart procedure.

I had never been victim of a real surgery before. Yes, near-countless Cardioversions and a couple of catheter-based procedures, but those were simple. Simple and the toughest parts were some general discomfort—in stark contrast to real pain—and some concern about the anesthetics.

My experiences with pain were limited, but I did not like them. I broke my big toe as a kid. Of course everyone stubs toes—that's half the fun of being a kid! This one though cracked that sucker *the long way*. It hurt a lot, and there was nothing we could do for it. Zach—I'm sorry. This happened on the afternoon of one of your birthday parties—I'm guessing you were five or six years old, and I know I howled like a little girl in front of all your non-girl friends.

Beyond the terrible toe trauma, most of my pain was self-inflicted. Killer hangovers in my foolish younger years. Sprawling and violent ski crashes, both on water and on ice, and two years in orthodontia. Technically that was not self-inflicted, but I allowed it to happen, month after month, and I still hold myself responsible for not putting my foot down in protest (and, I promise, I never fantasized about driving that foot's sharp heel down through the delicate bones of that doctor's instep). Maybe I never had then, as a teenager, but apparently now I do hold that grudge and hang on to that decades-old desire.

Small potatoes, of course, and the real Idaho Special was that I would not have any grasp of the concept of real pain.

Cracked ribs are painful. A pinch in the side is tough. It seems like an acute-type pain there. The concept of a sternum-division is so nebulous that I could not fathom, and certainly could not discern the difference, or try to weigh the options. In my heart of hearts, I felt that if they had to cut, if they had to cut anywhere, I might as well let them have the full access. Again—this did not come into conversation with this first surgical interview, but it was in the back of my head. And in the side of my head was this silly little aversion to a slit between my ribs. Maybe too many hard-boiled detective novels describing the tough damage a knife can wreak when properly inserted into the gristly tissue between the natural guardians of our most critical organs.

Strangely, overall the concept of pain (nor, more significantly, recovery) never weighed into the equation. The only hint I had was from my buddy in an almost-giveaway line when first mentioning the mysterious Maze Procedure: "You're young, and strong. You could handle it (*now*, as opposed to decades from now)."

So maybe my lack of cognizance or care about pain is a reasonable excuse for not digging deeper into the whats and the hows in this initial consultation. And maybe it was the fact that it happened fast: a short, six-month honeymoon with Tikosyn, a flurry of phone calls with my primary EP after that drug fell out of favor, his "call the surgeon" response, and an almost-immediate appointment. All of a sudden I was looking at major surgery.

I tried to maintain some perspective through this process, but it almost seemed that the more research I did, even anecdotally, led to more consternation than not. My dog and I had a very nice conversation with some neighbors one afternoon. Mr. Neighbor had had a "four-way" years ago. By his description, the entire process was traumatic, starting with his regular cardiologist's check-up. That appointment revealed an immediate need. Immediate as in: "would you like to call your wife and have her bring a bag, or should we just start now, sir?"

My neighbor was sorry my saga was continuing, but I should look at the bright side—at least it was not life threatening, and especially that I had already had the "surprise" part of it. Years ago, and that was really pretty mild, comparatively-speaking.

And then he mentioned the pain. He's quick to show his forearm scars (procedurally, they harvest similarly-sized blood vessels from the forearms, and legs, in order to place them in replacement of the clogged ones near the heart). His arms hurt the worst. He still shuddered a little as he described it. So again, good for me—no ancillary cutting or harvesting necessary!

And then they broached a subject that had not crossed my mind, at all. Depression.

Depression? According to my neighbors, it was tough. And when it is tough on him, it is of course tough on her. Years later they were of course smiling and healthy now, and therefore eager to share with me. But it was tough for me to imagine. First, I had not known this couple then, and secondly, yes, they seem totally healthy.

But Mr. Neighbor pontificated that he thought it had something with the heart being, literally and physically, out of its element. Apparently there can be a physiological link between body and mind. When the body's engine is out of sorts, the mind notices, and recognizes that something is not right.

I had not considered that, in the abstract nor certainly in the detail. While they were not going to remove my heart and replace bits and pieces from the parts bin, there may be some logic to the fact that my half-mast heart had been affecting, or could affect my outlook on life for the coming months.

My neighbor remarked that the recovery was very tough and that probably self-perpetuated his depression. When you can't do something, or do it well, or when you can't do *anything*, it's a significant weight on a previously-active person. And actually, active or not—it can weigh upon a person who has previously been simply self-sufficient.

Hmm…more food for thought. As if it's not enough to consider: what, where, by whom, when, should I even bother, how do I plan for day-to-day, long-term absence, it is worth it, etc.?

———

So, needless to say, after a best-in-class initial consultation, we had to muddy the water. We sought another opinion. And apparently this is not a unique concept. It's a widely-used step in the process, but I was more than a little surprised to see it on another local hospital's website: "Second Opinions Here" right in their Cardiac Expertise propaganda!

No—it is not my preference to do medical research on the Internet, but it sure is an easy place to start. Look up a phone number, read some bios on the docs, and then pick up the phone. I had planned on hours and hours—wrangling records from my current provider, paving the way with my insurer, etc. I was wrong, though. Seeking the "Second Opinion" was like hitting the "Easy" button.

———

Within a couple of days we had an appointment at another terrific local hospital, with a renowned cardiology department.

Also another very fine physician, and reassuring all around. There was less eager bluster and less scribbling on exam room paper, but it still made us feel good. And that is part of the conundrum. Nearly all modern medicine is darn close to miraculous in what they can perform. And at top-rated hospitals, the line between one provider and another is no more than razor-thin. How much time and effort should we put in, trying to find that exact silver bullet? In all likelihood, 98% of my options will yield a similar, if not completely satisfactory result.

But it is MY health. And it is MY heart, which is a pretty critical part of MY overall well-being and longevity. Forever. And for that reason, no stone should go unturned. We should be clad in Kevlar confidence that a particular procedure is the right one, at the right time, and performed by the right professional.

My second opinion had nothing to cause red flags to wave, but at the same time angels did not sing from the heavens in unison. Toward that, this particular physician was a generalist, who then had to refer me to a potential surgeon. His time, and his effort in the surgical referral were helpful, if only that going through the process and looking at options made me feel better at the end.

This surgical referral was so efficient that the cardiologist called me directly that afternoon. He had spoken with the surgeon already, and he would be happy to speak with me. The catch was that he was on vacation, and I was about to be. The surgeon asked this generalist: "Is the patient an okay guy? If so, go ahead and give him my cell. number." I was glad that I had at least passed the "crackpot" screening, although I can understand his trepidation. There are plenty of us out there, who do and would obsess, worry, and ultimately abuse a direct hotline to an expert.

So, this doctor called me back from the backwoods of Alabama, where he was visiting his parents' summer place. And I was driving north to Heather's sister's wedding in Milwaukee. While our conversation was fruitful, it was a far cry from spending an hour together in close consultation. A fine line perhaps between responsiveness to a patient in need, or eagerness to pluck a pigeon. I will admit it—if this practice had deferred me even a few days, let alone a customary few weeks, until I could be wedged into the surgeon's schedule, it would have soured me. As it was, I felt appreciative of the phone consultation, but also a little leery of its salesmanship—"don't worry, I know how to do this, and we'll see it once we get in there, and we can make it work, and we have the resources of this great university hospital behind us"...in between dropping the call three times because I was on the interstate and he may or may not have been on a boat.

Welcome to Rochester

As (I) PREDICTED, the second opinion only diluted the clarity offered by the first opinion.

The good news was that a tiebreaker was only one opinion away (never mind the fact that it's not a simple binary choice—much like determining someone's sex nowadays).

It had been no more than a week from the EP throwing up his hands to the first surgical consultation all the way through the second opinion. In that week, though, I think the situation's significance was sinking in.

It is MY health. And it is MY heart, which is a pretty critical part of MY overall health. Forever.

It was time to call in the big guns. I asked a close family friend for a referral to the Mayo Clinic, and within two hours my phone identified a call from the 507 area code.

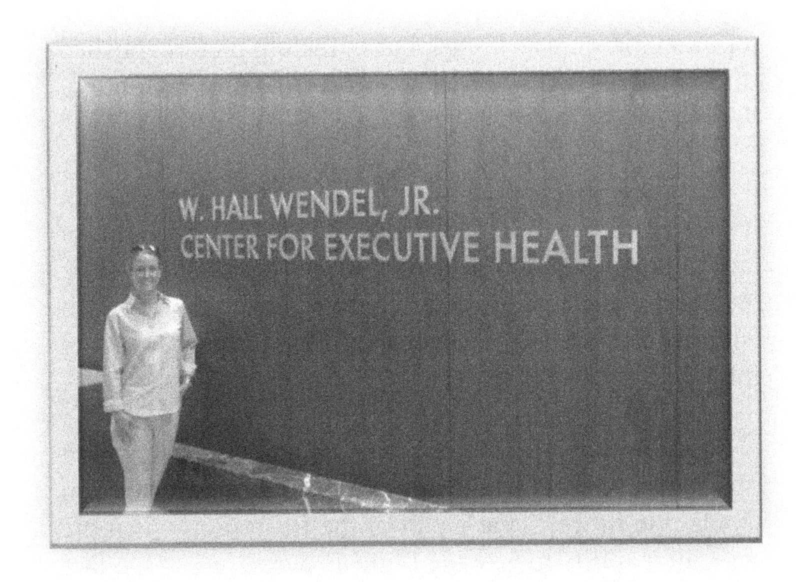

One concept sticks with me as I recall our personal journey, but the details escape me. That is probably a good thing. I think it was maybe because the "Tikosyn sucks" moment was such a surprise to us, and then we immediately lurched into "surgery" mode, it was stressful. Very stressful, and my wife and I handle stress differently. That is often a good thing, but in this case, the seemingly simple task of choosing the what, who, and where was awful.

I know we were thankful to have the opportunity to discuss my case with Mayo, but it was also not the right out of the box cure-all I might have hoped.

I'm probably responsible for the bulk of our stress. Initially I was against the second opinion, because in my head we had nowhere to go but down. That second opinion did muddy things, but in the big picture, pushed the needle back significantly toward our first option. Good, simple, huh? Nope.

As the concept coalesced for me, I probably did not communicate it well, and things did devolve into a bit of an unintentional competition. I only mention that here because I am sure we are not the only family with slightly differing viewpoints or decision-making processes.

Heather has been my staunch ally through thick and thin during my time at Provider A. And there have been some thin times. That's part of the frustration—is it the overall inability to provide finite answers, or is it the fact that we got a grumpy nurse one day who complicated one appointment? Probably combinations of both. Every month. And that made me feel I had to defend Provider A to my wife. Part of it is that I have felt comfortable overall, and another part of it is simple trepidation toward change.

Heather has a history (albeit not with the cardiology department) at Provider B. A mixed-bag history, but a history nonetheless. As we sought a consultation there, I think she was advocating there—partly out of "grass is greener" optimism, and partly out of her frustration at Provider A.

Both perspectives are valid. But they did not make the process any easier for us. By the time I made the Mayo call, I was planning on taking the consultation trip myself. That would have been a bad idea. Yes, it might have been simpler. Hell—there's no *might* about it—it would have been a thousand percent simpler (in the short-term). I could have left at the drop of a hat, I could have taken copious notes...and then come home and have had to explain my decision and troubleshoot pitfalls...for the rest of my life.

As it turns out, Heather alerted me to the folly of that thought, and "we" decided that of course she would join me on that trip. And yes, of course I'm glad—especially because the early bloodletting was an important part of our consensus of opinion once we did hit upon the solution. It took us a couple extra days to plan and to get out of town—dog/house sitter, time off work, etc.—but it was worthwhile.

———

From that first phone call welcoming me to the Mayo Clinic, Swiss watch makers should all be jealous. The representative described the process, and I was immediately left with some work to do following her clear instructions. Most of my work was at home, as Heather and I had agreed to seek the third opinion there and then wrangled with how and when to get there. As I called back with my open window of dates, my representative already had everything loaded and ready to go. Before hanging up (and they always answer the phone, and the person you are seeking is always available), she had emailed me an itinerary.

My name was on it, spelled correctly, and the dates accurately corresponded to what we had discussed. While on the phone, my representative described that she had already cleared my pathway to Dr. N, who is spectacular. He was to be my alpha and my omega. Now, she may not have known a cardiologist if he hit her in the funny bone, but from my end of the phone, it sounded like she had personally screened all potential physicians in the 24 hours since her first call to me.

I began poring over the itinerary, and was pleased to have such a remarkably efficient overview at my fingertips. It was planned by the minute, and told me which building, which floor, and at which desk to report. It was amazing.

And as we progressed through that first day on campus, I stayed on, or ahead of (!) schedule. Think about it—where, in modern life, does a schedule actually work? Let alone over the course of meeting several different providers, in several different buildings, and with multiple tests built in—some taking three minutes, and some taking more than an hour. Unbelievable, but that is a particularly good example of Mayo's classic professionalism and efficiency. Maybe a Mussolini of the Midwest was on their planning committee.

In his memoir *A Lucky Life Interrupted,* Tom Brokaw describes: "The (Mayo) Clinic is a patient-friendly system with expansive lobbies and sunny solariums as a welcome retreat for patients facing the unknown or a defined condition that has no good outcome. The real genius is in the management of every patient who comes through the doors. A Saudi prince may get more personalized attention than a Wisconsin schoolteacher, but both will be the central figure in a system where all of the attending physicians and technicians on the case are sharing the same information and constantly communicating with one another about what's best for the patient. Sounds logical, no?"

———

Every Mayo staffer carried themselves as utmost professionals. But more importantly, as *caring* professionals.

At my first appointment I was checked in by an aide in shirt and tie under a smock. He was polite and cordial and efficient. A real Girl Friday. As Friday was running through the questionnaire, I was nervous. It felt like this was the pinnacle of my journey. And I damned well better know my stuff, and certainly not waste the doctor's time. It's not easy to keep all these appointments on time, you know.

And yet, upon Dr. N's entrance to the consultation room, it was like meeting a dignitary, and frankly, he made Heather and me feel like dignitaries ourselves. He made sure to greet us both, taking time to listen to our names, and our story. In retrospect, he can of course learn a lot about a potential patient that way, but it is a learned method. And not an easily-learned one.

I think that is important to point out because in this nebulous world of arrhythmia, persistent or paroxysmal can mean vastly different things across different patients (and even physicians).

Was I truly afflicted? Could I tell the difference? Was I doing everything I could to understand, fix, or even just mitigate the problem? Was I seeking attention? How did it all make me feel? How did it make my wife feel?

Could the doctor see a commitment in me, equal to his commitment to practicing his craft expertly? I know that sounds high-handed of me, but it is indicative of the audition feeling I had before the meeting.

I don't mean to suggest that there is any capricious selectivity in the medical profession. But I do feel strongly that this needs to be a two-way street. When making an appointment with a medical professional, I am seeking their expert services. Their service is based upon years of education, which allows for high levels of deductive reasoning and analytics as tools to help my condition. If I do not provide them with good information, I am wasting everyone's time and money. To say nothing of potentially impugning the physician's reputation, standing in his profession, and ability to make a living. Some of this may be hyperbole, but I have a feeling, with the current state of our medical industry, physicians need to be cognizant of issues like this. While baristas and other self-proclaimed underemployed across the country can capriciously renege on their student loans, it would not bode well for the professional progress of a member of this select fraternity to do so.

———

So, while I was nervous and apprehensive, confident and eager all at the same time, this felt like a moment of truth.

Professional and caring are the two words I can best use to describe Dr. N. It felt almost like a strange stitch in time, because the entire time we were "on campus," it was clear that things were moving on a well-calculated schedule. I almost expected the doctor to march me doubletime through a handful of questions, after pronouncing that he's "got exactly twelve and a half minutes," or something like that.

In actuality, it was the exact opposite. The good (or great!) doctor was there, in the room, intensely, and with nothing else on his mind. He was concentrating on my case—my care, actually—and took time to get to know Heather and me. I realize I sound fawning. That is my memory. At the time, it was cordial, professional, and the best use of more than an hour throughout my entire saga.

He was intense, but also cognizant that we are all human beings. Even he, even me. His sole focus was to figure out a path to make me (and Heather) feel better. He was not concerned with hitting his lunch hour, nor, frankly, with impinging upon his colleagues' schedule. Once he felt good about where we were, and his initial analysis of the situation, he pronounced that I had to go see Dr. S. And while he uttered that sentence, he was simultaneously dialing the exam room phone and his cell. phone.

Dr. S is the "THE Rhythm Guy." And as such his time is in high demand. Whomever Dr. N tracked down on whichever phone—I couldn't quite tell, offered that Dr. S was in surgery through the morning and in consultation or rounds through the afternoon.

Dr. N did not have to push. It seemed to be clear that if he was making this call for a consultation, it was important. And it was—for that particular patient in front of him at that particular moment. Dr. S's office offered that he would be happy to see me that evening. Would 6:45 work for me? Um, yes, of course. We were happy to work around his schedule. Of course.

Even though nothing had been decided at this initial meeting with Dr. N, we already felt a thousand percent better. It was a huge relief already that I had been taken seriously, that this doctor took decisive action, and that we felt valued throughout.

While Dr. N was friendly throughout, I had been reticent to make small talk. But near the end, I had to ask. We have some good friends from the Middle East, and I was close to giggling at times throughout the meeting, because the good doctor's accent was nearly identical. My friend is terrifically intelligent, but also averse to doctors, so it was comical hearing high-level, empathetic medical talk from the same voice. The doctor hails from a neighboring republic in the Fertile Crescent. The accent was uncanny.

We walked back to the hotel instead of taking the shuttle. Then wandered back into downtown and had an early dinner, and then took the shuttle over to the other campus. It was a beautiful summer's day, made better by this burden of "making the cut," so to speak, having been lifted from our shoulders already.

———

Dr. S was clearly tired—he had probably already *worked* twelve hours at least, but he did not let on as such. There was zero pretense, and his focus was solely on this patient, this customer.

It felt like a brief consultation because his "analysis" was very brief. All told, we spent probably an hour and a half with him. His analysis was five minutes' worth of conversation, and then a grueling physical component. He felt my pulse in each wrist, and then led me down the hall to a stairway. I was to climb one flight of stairs twice. I did so, and he felt my pulse again, in each arm. I believe his quick exam showed that my heart reacted normally to very light activity. His summation then was that I was a "normal, otherwise healthy 42-year-old male."

I have a feeling that Dr. N had filled him in on the more particular particulars. They do their homework, and do not enter into diagnoses or plans lightly. I know Dr. N had scanned my history thoroughly, and internalized each and every procedure.

———

Dr. S Mayo Clinical Note: 6/25

HISTORY OF PRESENT ILLNESS ***Delightful 42-year-old male here with his wife.*** *He has been troubled with atrial fibrillation now for a few years. In May three years ago, he presented with atrial fibrillation, fatigue, and rapid ventricular response. He had a TEE-guided cardioversion, and at that time, a small atrial septal defect measuring 3 x 4 mm with left-to-right shunting was found. Because of other documented recurrences and cardiac MRI that showed moderate right ventricular enlargement. He had and a 13 mm Amplatzer ASD occluder device placed. The procedure was without complication.* ***For the past two and a half years, he has had recurrences of atrial arrhythmias which have included atrial flutter as well as atrial fibrillation. He has had previous attempts at rhythm control with flecainide at 100 mg twice daily, caval tricuspid isthmus ablation, and dofetilide at 500 mcg twice daily. Despite these he has had recurrence of symptomatic atrial fibrillation and now is seeking opinion for further management.*** *He has been anticoagulated with apixaban. He has visited with physicians who have recommended either a classic cut and sew surgical maze procedure or a more minimally invasive mini-Maze type of procedure. He met with Dr. N earlier and now comes for further discussion.* ***His symptoms include a significant drop in his quality of life and effort tolerance.*** *He is aware of, but not particularly troubled, by the palpitations. He has no history of hypertension, diabetes, previous stroke, or TIA.*

PHYSICAL EXAMINATION General: He is alert, well oriented. He is thin. Heart: There is no chest deformity. His metacarpals are normal. Heart rate is in the 60s with occasional ectopy, and the heart rate response to a brisk hall walk and a one-flight stair climb were normal. There is no evidence of heart failure.

IMPRESSION/REPORT/PLAN #1 Symptomatic atrial fibrillation with prior Amplatz closure of an ASD. I had a lengthy discussion with the patient and his wife with regard to treatment options. In terms of invasive and surgical options, I described methods for ablating atrial fibrillation, including pulmonary vein isolation, linear ablation, ablation in and around the right superior vena cava, and other triggers for atrial fibrillation. In terms of technical details with his Amplatzer in place, I described approaches of going around, including through the superior limbus above the Amplatzer device, retrograde approaches to isolating the pulmonary veins or ablating triggers, and percutaneous epicardial approaches. With regard to surgical approaches, I distinguished between minimally invasive approaches and the cut and sew Maze procedure. We discussed the risks, benefits, and details of each of these. I briefly also described pacemaker-based approaches. He asked me what the most definitive procedure would be without the need of permanent pacing and pacemaker dependence, and I told him it would probably be the cut and sew Maze procedure. We also discussed the fact that ablation is possible after a Maze procedure and vice versa. They will think of these options and discuss with Dr. N before proceeding.

———

While Dr. S' physical "examination" took maybe four minutes (but I know it felt interminable to Heather when he led me out of the room by my wrist and measured my pulse as I walked the hallway and two flights of stairs), the meeting was thorough. We (yes, we) talked through my history, and its ups and downs and my according and mounting worry. And *frustration,* of course—let's not lose sight of that watchword.

We discussed the rationales for each step to-date, and then went into the options moving forward. And there were options—a concept unembraced by the other surgeons I had met with at home.

Again—I did not let pain weigh on my decision. Maybe that is indicative of how fed up I was with the marathon that I could not run.

Working through the options, the doctor was like an efficient and purposeful attorney. He led me down the road, and never forced anything upon me. We knew what was coming, and as Heather and I looked at each other, I proclaimed that I felt good about my prospects with the Cut-and-Sew Maze surgery.

As I consider months later, I realize it was a fine line—he was not going to let me totally self-diagnose or claim to know my best course of action. But, he very clearly wanted me to understand the options and feel good about a collective decision point. And that's what it was.

He was earnest in his response—he thought that was the best plan for me, and he was encouraged that it would serve me well in the long run.

We again looked at each other recognizing relief, as I worked to formulate my next question. I knew in my head where I wanted to have this surgery, but I also absolutely needed to consider Heather's well-being and her burden. I began clumsily recounting that I was probably comfortable with some of my options at home—I appreciated the great efforts of Dr. S and Dr. N, and needed their counsel a little further. I had to be concerned about the added logistical headaches of a road game.

Before I could get any further, Dr. S took over. He had led us through a consultative process and we all felt good and were on the same page. Now, however, medical expertise was paramount. There were no two ways about it—if I was to have a Maze Surgery, I was going to do it at Mayo, and there was one guy who was going to do it: Dr. H. Dr. S would arrange it, but he would hear nothing of pursuing alternative providers. He said it more nicely than that, but it was clear that there was no wiggle room. And that itself was the best relief.

We had a plan. We fully agreed on the what, the where, and I was fortunate to get the best possible who.

If he were to have an ablation procedure, I told him that either myself or one of my colleagues would be happy to do the procedure here at Mayo Clinic Rochester. If he did decide on this surgical approach, he asked for a recommendation. and I recommended if Dr. N were in agreement, Dr. H for the Maze procedure.

Pre-Op to Post-Op

DURING THE COUPLE weeks post-consultation and pre-surgery, I received more advice than I could ever use. Some was helpful. Most, of course, was not. I believe all was well-intentioned.

Almost immediately upon our return home, I had a call from Mayo: "Dr. H could do your procedure on July 28—will that work for you?" "Um yes, of course!" Who was I to bicker about the schedule? Having it scheduled was almost as much relief as confirming the plan of action.

Having a couple weeks preceding the surgery was useful. One week would probably have been okay for me to plan, but I know the larger window was helpful for Heather. And I wasn't going to argue, especially as she was going to shoulder all of the burden (once I was in, out, and recovering). Before then, however, the fortnight led to some restlessness on my part. And probably some self-pity.

That's where some of the non-helpful advice came in, and was frustrating. Lots of people had opinions, and one was from a family member's date. I think I had met her once or twice but she immediately passed on her significant concern about depression—did the doctors offer any counseling for me? What was I going to do? I surely needed to be worried about this! She was suggesting books I should read, and strongly recommended that I consult a therapist before, and set appointments for afterwards. Wrong-o.

I had not given that any thought—even after the well-meaning, convivial, and concerned conversation with my neighbors a couple weeks earlier. I thought his situation was markedly different from mine, and I totally understood his concern (of his own situation). Mine was vastly different—it was not a surprise, not an emergency, and was going to finally provide me some much-needed and long-term relief.

So, I was restless. I continued to exercise, when in sinus rhythm. And when I was able, I did so strenuously. I was concerned about falling out of shape in my recovery. In retrospect, I should not have worried about being in shape at all, and I should have concentrated on putting on some weight beforehand. But what did I know? Blissfully, very little—I was to be in some very capable hands.

I made business plans, I made personal plans, and I did what I could to be extra helpful to Heather. I probably did also feel like a lame, lame duck. I might have had an extra cup of leaded coffee or a diet Coke, and I probably had a more frequent cigar than usual—what's the difference now? All told, I don't think I was a particularly ill-humored pre-patient…(but I was certainly peevish enough within my own head).

———

The day arrived. The travel day, anyway. My surgery was scheduled for a Tuesday, but I had to show up for tests and whatnot first thing Monday morning. So we loaded the large SUV to the gills, and drove north. My Mom met us in Rochester, and we enjoyed some social time and meals, including a "last supper" on Monday night.

During the down times on Monday I tried to schedule my post-op appointment at home. Tried to being the operative (so to speak) words here. Caution to future patients—if you are having an off-campus surgery, make sure there is good communication between providers. My home team was going through a computer conversion (about their fourth in my time there, it felt), and they could not even return phone calls, let alone schedule anything. And I was in dreamland hoping they would schedule per my ideal date—I had aimed for September 7th, which would have been too-optimistically early, anyway. I made one more attempt while we were at lunch on Monday the 27th, and offered, in a voicemail message that they would need to call my wife to confirm, as I might not be available. And then I forgot about it. Good for me, bad for Heather. I did not leave explicit directions asking her to ride herd on it. And we didn't revisit it until we were headed home on Thursday August 6th.

———

Monday the 27th was filled with tests and pre-surgery appointments with my various team members. Strangely enough, I had assumed (before I received my detailed itinerary) that we would have had a grand meeting around a conference table with my "team." That was not the case. Everything was of course well-planned and timed, but all sequential and separate. Blood, EKG, Echo, etc., and then physician meetings. These, I think had one simple purpose—to monitor my state of mind perhaps to ensure I had not totally lost it since my last visit. And more importantly, simply to make me feel better about the big day to come. As I think back with vast experience now, we covered nearly no new territory, but our meetings with my close personal friends Drs. N and S did make me feel wholly comfortable going in—and more importantly, Heather was further reassured.

The one new meeting was with the inestimable surgeon himself, Dr. H. We spent a short amount of time with a clerk, updating my particulars (never mind the fact that the real data was being beelined from all corners of the hospital in real-time as tests were collected). And then a dashing young woman swooped into the consultation room. By her air of officialdom and quick effectiveness, I thought she might have been the hospital's COO, reporting straight to me from an all-staff medical summit. But perhaps more effectively, she was the surgeon's Physician Assistant, and yes, all things did seem to revolve around her (in a good way). She was like a medical incarnation of my wife—I was to be in great shape, they were both looking out for me!

We had a substantial conversation with her, furthering the feelings of faith. And then the surgeon—pardon me, The Surgeon—joined us. This was a quick part of the meeting. He did a very brief visual exam of my mental state (by boring straight through my eyeballs and into my soul with his questions), covered his legalities, and then asked if we had any questions. Mercifully he did not ask if we had any "final" questions.

Despite his giving the aura that we should not have any questions—the superstar PA should have covered *everything*—we felt obliged to pretend to participate. So Heather, buttoning everything up, as is her way and right, realized she was still a little unclear about a bit of logistics: "so, are you going in the side of the ribcage, or will you crack him open in the middle?"

"We will, yes, *divide the sternum.*" And that's about it for that meeting. We had learned a medical term (euphemism?), and learned to appreciate that The Surgeon's talents are quite specific indeed.

The PA picked us up, figuratively, completed the nuts and bolts of the meeting, and the feelings of respectful bonhomie were restored.

———

Dr. H Mayo Clinical Notes: 7/27

IMPRESSION/REPORT/PLAN The patient is a 42-year-old man from Kansas who has symptomatic paroxysmal atrial fibrillation and flutter. *His symptoms began three years ago. During initial evaluation he was found to have a small atrial septal defect. This was closed with an occluding device, but atrial arrhythmias persisted and he then underwent ablation of atrial flutter. The patient has had recurrent episodes of atrial fibrillation and has tried multiple medications including metoprolol and flecainide.*

Because the ASD device is in place he is not a candidate for repeat atrial fibrillation ablation and he comes now for consideration of a Maze procedure. I met with the patient and his wife to discuss operation. I explained the procedure and the anticipated recovery both in the hospital and at home. ***I emphasized that the chance of success is 90% but not 100%. Risk of operation is 1% or less. The patient would like to proceed.***

INFORMED CONSENT I discussed the situation in detail with the patient including diagnosis, pathology, planned operation, objective, risks, benefits, alternatives, and the necessity of other members of the surgical team participating in the procedure. Risks include but are not limited to death, stroke, infection, bleeding, myocardial infarction, and potential need for blood transfusion. Advanced directives regarding hospitalization following surgery were discussed, and all agree that we would resuscitate if the need arose. The patient understands the uncertainties and wishes to proceed. All questions were answered as completely as possible.

———

Probably the best part of the pregame was when I hit my window to call in and find out my "report time." While it felt a little frustrating beforehand that they could not commit to a scheduled time, I think I understand that a surgical schedule needs to be a little fluid—right up until fewer than twelve hours prior. The prescribed call-in time was while we were enjoying a wonderful walleye dinner. I watched the minutes tick by, and then, feeling a little bit like a participant in a Southwest Airlines check-in scramble, called the hotline. I plugged in my code, and jackpot! I was to be there at 5:45 am. Hallelujah. The waiting was the hardest part, and it grew increasingly tiring as we grew closer to the witching hour. And now fortunately, my hour was nigh. It worked great—we finished dinner, complete with a sampling of desserts, had a nice walk through downtown and back to the hotel, and I did not have extra time to fret.

The Layman's Description:

What is a "Maze Procedure?" I did not let the mechanics of the procedure enter into my decision to (follow the professionals' suggestions to) undergo it. I intentionally did not know—either before considering, or after committing.

If I did know, I would have done more than simply "fret."

Succinctly, the upper chambers of the heart are cut, and then sewn up, to create actual, flesh-and-blood scarring. This scar tissue interrupts errant electrical signals. Therefore, the heart relies only upon its intentional signals.

I describe it as the "mother of all open-heart surgeries" because it is traumatic, to the entire organ. As opposed to fixing a valve or four, or relieving a blockage—those are area-specific. In the Maze (named because it cuts a literal maze across the tissue, stopping straight-line signals), the entire thing is filleted and traumatized.

Right decision for me...but it's still too much information.

———

I took my last shower with the dreadful disinfectant soap, and turned in for a decent sleep.

The welcome pre-dawn alarm sounded, and I was packed and ready to go. I think I was even moderately patient as I waited for my mom and Heather in the hotel lobby. We did not leave as early as I had hoped, and that unfortunately made me a little crabby (couldn't have been the stress, though, huh?). Our early shuttle driver was efficient, though, and we did arrive on time (it's a four-minute trip—I really didn't need to pad it too much).

———

We walked into the well-lit and spotless lobby. Straight to the appropriate desk, with the airline analogy again apt. There were three "lanes," each marked with the arrival times. At 5:45, I was in Group A. But there was no one behind the counters!

Never to worry, the smiling clerks appeared at about 4:44:30, and cheerily welcomed the masses. It was an interesting crowd. Some full of nervous anticipation, perhaps like myself, and some (or most) clearly worn out, and some just plain anxious. And of course, cadres of loved ones. Several it seemed were in pajamas. Most were clutching tumblers of coffee, and a good number were carrying pillows and blankets. We were in it for the long haul.

I did not sharpen my elbows to get to the front of my 5:45 line, and it wouldn't have been unnecessary if I had tried. We were all cordial for the approximately three minutes we waited to clear the queue. After the orderly check-in at the desk, an actual Orderly escorted me back.

The prep room was tiny and busy. I was glad to have family with me…sort of. Their nervousness was oppressive. We did make nice small talk with the attendants, but it was not a tremendously social time—nor was there room for three Ehlerts in there, to say nothing of the medical professionals there to do their jobs.

I did put my foot down and ordered out all non-essential personnel once the razor specialist arrived. The guy was a professional, and so while his practice was not fun or pleasant for me, it was not painful. Only mildly uncomfortable, I took solace that this was a one-time deal for me; not so much for him. My chest had been shaved only two weeks prior, so that was not too bad. His orders, though, were: "neck to knees." The peanut gallery was not needed for this.

All told, there was almost no dead time. From the moment I checked in, things moved along officiously, but cordially. I think I had maybe ten minutes of clock-watching before I said my goodbyes and they wheeled me back, right at 7:00.

I don't think I was anaesthetized then, but I must have been nervous. I do not remember much beyond watching the clock click toward the top of the hour. I do not remember entering the operating theater. I do not remember the real flood of cold as the juice entered my arm, nor the elusive bliss as it took hold. I don't remember anything until waking up. And even that is hazy, at best.

———

Heather and my mom were brought in to see me when I was safely ensconced in the ICU. I was not awake. Heather to this day still remarks how great I looked. I know I had tubes and wires everywhere, but she was struck by how good my color was. They speak glowingly of their first meeting with my nurse: "Hi! I am Nurse G, and Dr. H did my open-heart surgery one year ago." (He then pulled down his green scrub top to reveal his 'zipper' scar). "See? Everything will be just fine!" Pretty cool way to alleviate their stress.

In the weeks and months of my recovery, the single most-heard comment was: "Wow, Adam—you look great. Your color is much better. You had really looked awful for a long time." "Um, thanks (I guess)." I clearly had not been able to see myself through others' eyes for a long period leading up to my surgery. I was bent on enjoying each "normal" beat I had, and I probably exercised too much, and I also was also foolishly worried about falling out of shape during several months of inactivity. So, I was too thin. I looked awful. My heart was not beating strongly or consistently. I know there was perpetual fatigue, worry and frustration hiding behind my eyes. I looked like a walking billboard for the word "pallor." So yes, even still-unconscious, tubes and wires everywhere, my first appearance was of healthy rosiness. This was my mom's first impression, and it makes me smile to hear of her relief at that moment.

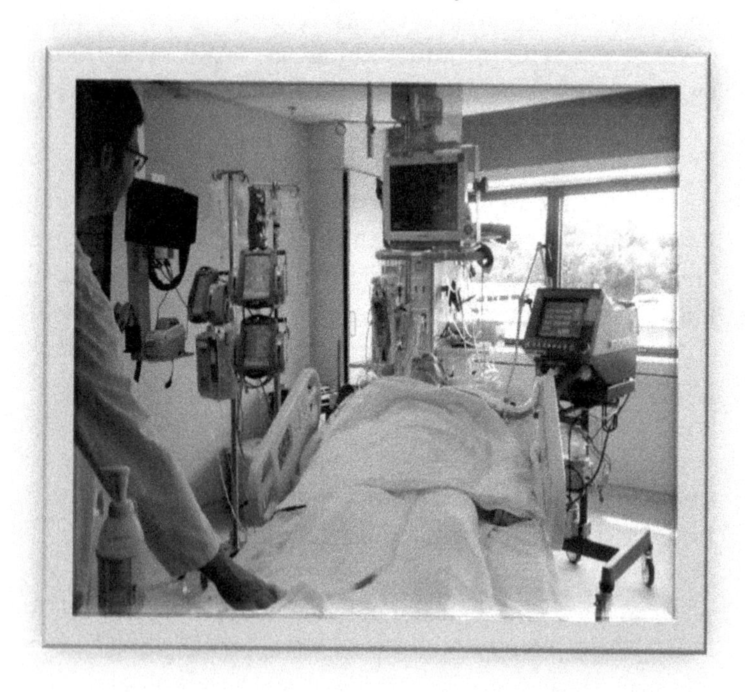

I awoke in the ICU. I do remember feeling glad to be awake, and glad to be there, but beyond that I did not feel good. And I apparently let that fact be known.

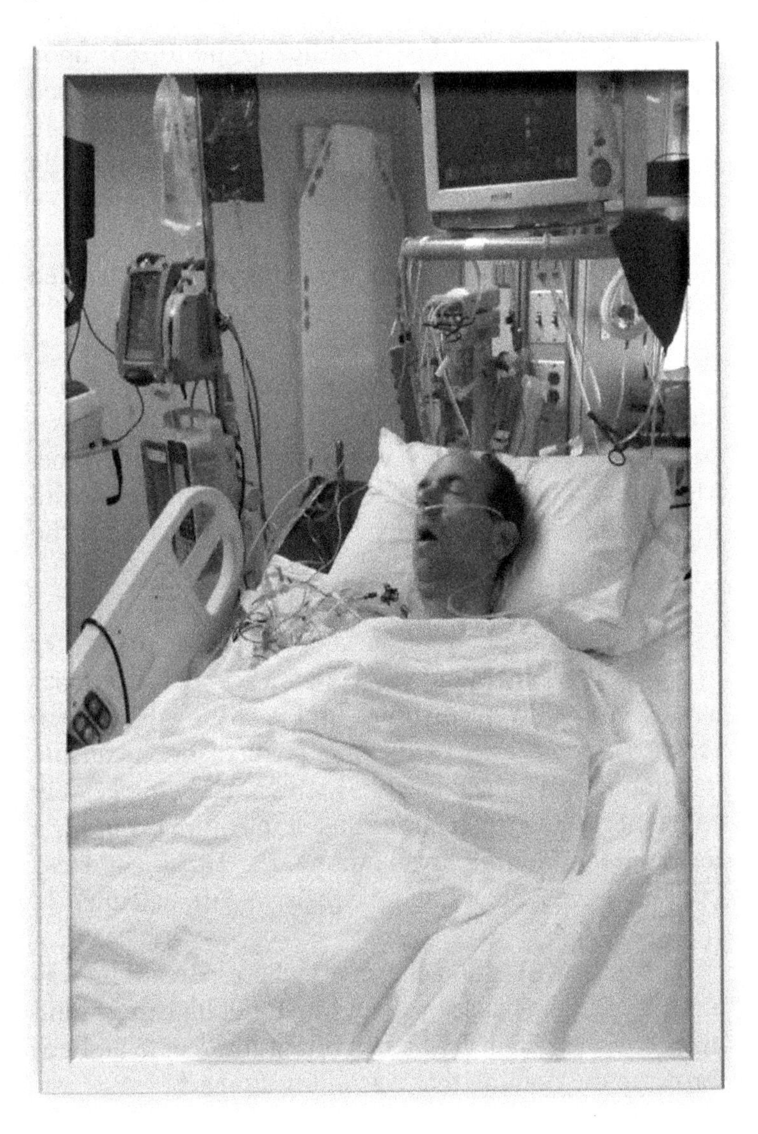

I vaguely remember meeting my nurse. He was a superstar, but details of that initial meeting are fleeting (to me, anyway). My nurse was insistent that the ladies had time to track down a late lunch, and he would take care of everything. Most specifically, he took it upon himself to remove my breathing tube. In his esteemed opinion, I was young and strong, and should not need it. It was only going to make me miserable—especially upon its removal.

The onlookers didn't want to see that, so they scuffled off in search of sandwiches (or smoothies?).

I guess I was almost conscious enough to take direction. He told me to breathe out as strongly as I could, and he apparently removed the breathing tube. Mercifully, I do not remember it, and I am thrilled he did it when he did. Especially because as I came to, the nausea was battling the pain for top billing.

I vaguely remember the direction to press the plunger in my hand every ten minutes for pain relief. I remember having zero concept of time—did each breath take ten seconds or ten years? I remember being distinctly unable to communicate this concern. I remember being acutely concerned about my nausea. Just a few minutes in (or a few hours—I don't know), I threw up. Thank goodness I did not have a breathing tube there to suffocate me.

The pain was a dull ache, everywhere. Breathing was a chore. But the nausea was awful. It felt like hours (and maybe it was?) that I was struggling to breathe and not throw up the nothing that was in my stomach.

I don't really recall the specifics of pain. Just the persistent nausea. I do not like feeling nauseated, and avoiding any flare-up of that was taking all of my concentration. For what felt like weeks.

It probably wasn't that long, but I do understand that I did not eat for at least a couple/few days. I was paranoid, and my providers were ultimately not happy about it. But I'm getting ahead of myself.

———

In those first several hours, I was struggling to know up from down. I vaguely remember meeting my nurse. I recall, very happily, that my mother and my wife were in the room when I awoke. It felt like an enormous room, dimly lit and quiet as a tomb, save the whisper of the machines near my bed.

But as big as the room was, there was only one chair for a visitor. Heather appropriately gave the chair to my mom. It might also be that Heather doesn't sit, or does not sit well.

I could not see my mom, as "the chair" was behind me, over my left shoulder. But I knew she was there. I also knew Heather was there. She, God bless her, is intense. And takes no guff—especially from me. Not even when I am not me.

What I recall was being wholly uncomfortable. And Heather looked uncomfortable and angry and restless. I can appreciate all that. They had a long, stressful day. I think my mom was off and on asleep in the visitor's recliner. Heather does not sit, nor certainly recline.

So, she hovered. At least that's what it felt like to me. She was circling left and right, arms crossed, glaring down at her incapacitated husband.

I remember struggling to form the words in my head. And then really struggling to get them out of my mouth. And yet I still fumbled the delivery. The clumsiness was: "It does not help me feel better with you inspecting me like I'm a zoo animal on display."

Somehow that did not go over well. To her credit, I think she gathered her things and her wits, and left the room without pointing out the folly of my words.

The irony is that I went out of my way to be kind to, and appreciative of, each and every person who touched me. And maybe that effort is part of what drove her, appropriately, nuts. I was so kind and thankful…to all except the most important person.

I know my exhausted mother stayed with me in the room throughout the afternoon and evening. Heather walked around and cooled off, and called my dad to offer him an update. I believe her exact words were: "He looks great. I know he's fine because he's an ass." Concise.

My dad had planned to come to Rochester for a few days, but not right away—by my account, I did not need extra people hanging around staring at me while I was incapacitated. I thought I planned that well. To comfort Heather, he came down that first night, took her to dinner, and then drove back to the Twin Cities afterwards. The next day he packed a weekend bag and headed back to Rochester for a few days according to plan.

By my (cloudy) observation, my plan did work well. My mom really wanted to be there, even though I wasn't, and she did a great motherly job of exhausting herself with an abundance of worry and absence of sleep. Heather had to take care of herself, and prepare to take care of me. It was a good combination then to have my dad as Heather's entertainment and restaurant escort, and my mom as the mother.

———

I think I was in the ICU for three days. I remember very little detail. One I do recall was when the surgeon and his team swooped in to see me. It was at least my second day, and he was aghast that I had not been up and walking yet. I really felt bad, mentally and physically. I wanted to follow doctors' orders, I wanted to alleviate the stress my family may have been feeling because of my "slow" recovery, and most of all, I wanted the nausea to go away. As that was pervasive, I could not do anything. I couldn't breathe, although I do think I was already valiantly trying to be diligent with the "Inspirational Respirometer." I couldn't eat or consume anything beyond ice chips. And therefore, I certainly could not get my ass out of bed and do something constructive. I really wanted to please the doctor, and he was clearly displeased that I was still immobile.

———

On the fourth day I was released to "the floor," which is the cardiac recovery floor. I'm fairly certain I had not moved a muscle, except for some very weak breathing.

Because I was not eating, my recovery was like a North Korean missile—it wasn't getting off the ground.

———

Heather Nightingale, of course, came to my rescue. She and the nursing and medical staff were at their wits' end waiting for me to start eating. The early concern was: we know the hospital food is awful, but that's okay. It is nourishing, and, perhaps more importantly, bland—which is good because whatever he does wind up eating now, he will probably never want to eat again the rest of his life.

I even was feeling guilty. I'd hear the chorus (a veritable chorus of angels, as it were) exclaiming "He's got to eat!" It was a vicious cycle—without nourishment, I couldn't gain strength, and I also couldn't handle my potent pain meds any better than I had been. But being unable to handle them, I was still wracked with nausea.

After a while The Surgeon was beside himself, while standing beside my bed. He did not care what it was that I consumed—it just had to be *something.* And he was losing patience with the staff who were clearly incompetent in getting this through my thick head. Yes, I was right there hearing this. In corpus anyway, if not in mentis. And my guilt grew. Not enough for me to be able to bang down an entire cup of something as exotic as Jell-O, mind you, but guilty in the dark recesses anyway.

My mom and Heather had become regulars at a little hippie food place just across the street from whatever building I was in. I think they had been seeking salads, and light breakfasts. They had found a good place.

In exasperated consultation with the nurses, they were seeking something I would eat, and would want to eat, and might keep down. By now I was probably well past the actual nausea, but I was still clearly gun-shy. The "taste" of nausea was still with me, and even months and months later, the memory of that unpleasantness in my nose and the feeling it sends southward makes me shudder.

The Smoothie Girl was very helpful to Heather (I think they have a well-placed business, nourishing both patients and family members alike, day in and day out). She was suggesting Chia seeds and celery root, and God knows what else. Heather was of course very protective of me, and probably also concerned about my crabbiness. She knew I would notice Chia seeds, and probably not touch the damned thing. She knew she could sell ice cream or milkshakes to me all day long, but dairy was not going to be good for my uneasy innards.

So they hit upon the magic formula. Lots of fruit, maybe some vegetables—I don't know. And a secret ingredient not to be shared with me until months later:

tofu. It worked. I know I was leery and probably defensive but I ate the technicolor thing. And then I ate a couple or few more the next day. They were my salvation—my amateur nutritionists—and the smoothies both.

After a day and a half of smoothies and occasional pickings at hospital food, I was truly on the mend. I began eating nearly everything put in front of me. It started with lunch the next day. I picked at a few things, but ate a nice cup of what wanted to be chicken noodle soup. Something to augment my smoothie diet.

And then the real nourishment arrived. Some dear relatives made the trip from central Minnesota down to the southern part of the state. It was a several-hour trip for them, and it meant the world to us. She brought several wonderful things, but the only one I can remember is the real, hearty, homemade chicken noodle soup.

I felt the strength coursing through my veins. With each bite my physical and mental outlook surged. Thank you, Bob and Marilyn—your visit helped (both of us) tremendously. Very kind of you.

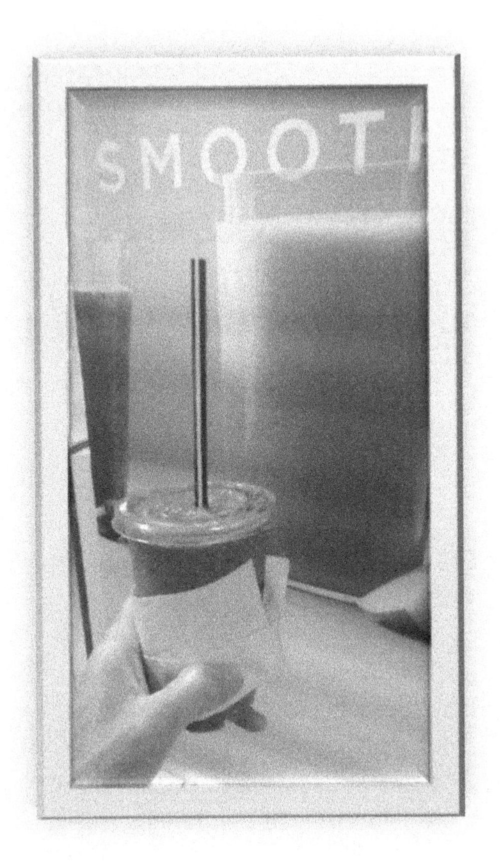

Smoothie update:

Heather loves telling her story of how she happened upon my magic elixir. And I never tire of thanking her for it. I have to hit the punchline, though. Several weeks later, as I was slowly becoming lucid in my home recovery, I looked at a credit card bill. There must have been a dozen of these $14.00 charges in downtown Rochester, MN. $14.00 a crack?!?!?! Had I known then (the tofu, OR the price), I never would have touched them. Strangely, I enjoy airport smoothies—perhaps the $9.00 price tag is comparatively palatable.

Good Provider, Bad Provider

I RECOGNIZE MY significant good fortune to have had my near-choice of providers.

Even before that, I am simply lucky to be in an area of excellent facilities and well-educated, enduring and unflappable healthcare providers. God bless Middle America! I did not walk into an Emergency Room and wait behind victims of violence, car crashes, drug overdoses, or Rahm Emmanuel-style errant gunplay. I never had to wait at all. I walked in, and attentive nurses, administrators, technicians and physicians were all at the ready to attend to me.

More significantly, our American system, while still insurer-saddled, is head and shoulders above the rest of the world.

Overall, I am thankful for the care I have received. Professionals in the industry have all invested heavily in themselves, and have devoted their lives to making mine better. They take on mountainous student loan debt, sacrifice time with family (often even avoiding the potential for a family until at a stable point in their career), and, with today's morass of regulation and liability this commitment to care does not even come with a guarantee of a viable profession and secure lifestyle.

Even in the best-case scenario, though, nothing is foolproof. One weak link can sour a patient's perspective. And that is a recurring theme.

A recent stay at my local institution came after a flurry of tests and interpretations of those tests, and resultant phone calls to and from me. It's not easy. It did happen fairly quickly, though, and I give my cardiology provider's practice credit on this one. Two days after wearing a Holter monitor, it showed some significant patterns (or, lack of patterns, as it were…) that required me to re-up on Tikosyn. The phone nurse was great with the presumptive, Option A or Option B close: "Mr. Ehlert, would you like to check in this afternoon, or tomorrow morning?"

So, I adjusted my professional and personal life, and planned to check in the next afternoon. I spent as much time at the office that morning as possible, raced home, packed an absolutely superfluous bag, and Heather handled my commute.

My "Admissions Clerk" was being trained. I can't complain about that—we all need to start somewhere. What I can and should complain about is the fact that her sole training was on the computer. Was there a patient in the room with her? She didn't know and she didn't care.

She would work through a few screens of information, mumbling to herself, checking my paper records and perhaps her system cheat sheet, and then roll away seeking her trainer. He'd come in and very expertly and officiously point to "click here, advance that screen there," and neither of them ever bothered to look to me, let alone look me in the eye while "communicating" with me. And upon culmination, she tried to rip some hair from my arm. I swear I am not a particularly hirsute person, nor am I particularly vain. But one simple step of crookedly attaching my wristband can lead to three and a half days of frustration.

Yes—continued reminder—one has to advocate for one's own position and care. I know I offended this poor clerk who was trying as best she could, and as well as she had been trained, but I quickly straightened the wristband myself before the glue fully cured. It was flat-out carelessness. She only barely reached over her desk and slapped it around my arm. Taking the time to do so carefully would have gone a long way.

I know I sound like a curmudgeon, but I am blaming it on four years of medical-industrial-complex-induced fatigue. I need a government program.

It really is unfortunate—here at a facility with all the resources in the world, they do not teach every clerk to care. And I'm not looking for a hug—in fact, that's the last particular thing I want—all I expect is someone to look me in the eye, welcome me, tell me what they are going to do and engage with me as they are doing it, and be proud of what "we" accomplish. It is training—you cannot count on common sense or human courtesy. Stepping away during the process because you need help is not the end of the world—simply sidling away, without communication is the end of the world, from the customer's (yes, *customer's)* perspective.

In this same mid-winter incursion, I continued to encounter, on a daily basis, both the bad and the good. The bad was the clerk who simply didn't know any better. Not a huge deal, but not a nice way to begin my stay. The tough point, is that the patient needs to maintain a sunny disposition, and essentially play a good *offense,* as opposed to being perpetually, guardedly, *defensive.* And it often is a fine line.

One of the RNs checking me in was familiar, having spent time in the Cardiac Rehab unit. Mercifully (for both of us, actually) she was one of the few that I didn't want to plant six feet under. In cognizance of that analogy, I hope her feeling to me was similar. She was one of the nurses at rehab who did not make my head explode. High praise, indeed.

She was perfectly fine—pleasant and helpful. But also hamstrung by an unwieldy system. She began getting ready to place my IV line, but the tech needed to draw blood right away. I pointed out this incongruity, but my logic was lost on the system. My nurse admitted, yes, they often can draw blood from the IV line, but in this case we needed time on my side—the sooner they tested the blood, the sooner they could administer the drug…and the sooner I eventually could get sprung. Got it.

So, the phlebotomist gouged my elbow, and then the nurse began my IV line. While trying to determine where, I did implore her to shave *more. Yes, more—no vanity here, especially when it comes time to remove the tape and bandages!* She obliged, sort of. She shaved more, but not enough to clear the area for the one bandage holding the IV in place. Yes—this becomes painful upon removal, but also, I think, is not totally effective.

They did rush off to get the blood in process of testing, which was nice. But, hours later, I was still cooling my heels. I checked in at 3:00 on a Thursday. With the hope then that I could get out before, at least, 3:00 on Sunday. That hope slowly waned, though, as it was past 11:00 before I had my first dose. The delay stemmed, partially, from my Magnesium shortage. They need me at 2.0, but I was underperforming at 1.9. So, they had to use that IV line. A couple hours' worth of a Magnesium drip…and then my results were at 2.1. Too much. No go, says Mission Control. By then I was good friends with my night nurse, and she did communicate well. She offered that she had to seek two doctors' override to administer the Tikosyn. And then it took multiple requests from the pharmacy (apparently not all of the system overrides reached them).

Her good communication (always welcome) was particularly nice because she understood the significance of timing. The normal statement is "three days" to load dofetilide. The real scenario is five doses. That was a nice reminder, and I was hopeful for a Saturday night release. But as the clock kept creeping, that potential was leaving the building, even as I was not.

The medication needs to be spaced 12 hours apart, with very little variation. So, with a first dose past 11:00 pm, my morning dose could be at 10:30, that night at 10:00. Then 9:30 the next morning, and 9:00 on Saturday night! The kicker, though, is that an EKG and a blood test is then needed two hours after the last dose. Sunday morning here I come.

I think I made it to "sleep" about 1:00 that first night. And sleep is in quotations because I am never really able to sleep while in the hospital. It's an awful combination—no energy, little motivation to do anything, a wholesale inability to concentrate even if I did want to do anything…and an absolute inability to get meaningful rest.

I'm going a long way in this vignette to show the huge impact that small things, good and bad, can have upon a patient's care. Simple communication within hospital departments is tough. That can all be alleviated by good communication to the patient. A smile, and genuine concern (or even feigned concern—I don't care!) goes even further.

———

WHAM! I'm half-asleep, and quickly less than half asleep when a bad provider slams in the room. And instantly I remember her from my last stay at The Restless Inn. I can smell her bad purple bubble gum from where she stands in the hallway after flinging the door open. My fears are confirmed when she takes her first self-respect-free shuffle/waddle step into my room. And before that step is halfway to its nine-inch stretch, she slams the overhead lights on. Without warning.

The last time she attacked me, I was in sorrier shape—a more significant case of round-the-clock persistent AFib. And perhaps it was my second night and I was more fatigued—I don't remember clearly. What I do remember is that she was so singularly untalented that I was nauseated. Yes, I had to call the nurse and ask for that medicine. I've said it before, I am a wimp—and I have passed out while needles are digging into my arm (see: Sarasota Memorial Hospital). There's not much room to fall when you're prone in a hospital bed, so I only lay there miserable waiting for the Alka Seltzer to take effect.

Anyway, this time I was stronger, apparently, and less affected by her indelicacies. It did hurt, though, and I resolved to two action points:

1) As good as many of my providers were, I always endeavor to thank them personally, and communicate praise to the hospital machine. In the case of this young lady, I would go out of my way to express that she clearly did not want to be here, and was not enjoying her job. I was fair and clear in my comment card, and not vengeful. But

I wasn't going to sit idly by while she inflicted her special brand of hell upon all who crossed her path.

2) If, I had occasion to be held captive by her again, I would quickly gather my 2:00 am wits, and refuse. I'll politely tell her that I needed the nurse's help, and that we would seek an alternative to her services. Again—a theme—advocate for yourself, even in a sleep-deprived state.

In my comment card I described her as a literal nightmare. The card I simultaneously completed was effusive in describing her next night's counterpart as a dream. Cynthia—yes, I remember her name—was just that.

She came into the room like a springtime breeze, and cheerily woke me, but just barely. She then introduced herself and described why she was there. She suggested I shield my eyes, as she couldn't do her job without turning on some lights. I don't know which lights she turned on (there are about five options—all lousy), but under Cynthia's delicate touch, the room gained a soft glow like it was a Lexus-designed dimmer. She asked which arm I preferred, and she went to work. As I was thanking her for being so caring and delicate…she was finished! I think I noticed her gentle pinch of my arm more than the needle. I was literally smiling as she whispered out of the room. I can imagine that is a very tough job, but wow—she took great pride in it, and took extra care to ensure my comfort. Gold-plated kudos for this woman.

You'll notice I did not say "young" woman. I think experience plays a lot into it. Cynthia had been around the block, and I think the Golden Rule was well-imprinted upon all members of her family. I imagine dozens of grandchildren clamoring for her attention. She knew what was important; both in life, and for little old me in room 225 at 2:00 on a February morning.

———

I mentioned the young-blood sucker's unpleasantness, and I also mentioned the seasoned Cynthia's expertise and pleasantness. And I've seen the best and worst of the spectrum. There is no single best scenario.

There's a typical cross-section of society at each position. It is funny, though—one can almost infer where these people are on the arc of their profession. The earlier-mentioned check-in clerk was probably north of fifty, and starting a new position—maybe a first professional one. She seemed okay on picking up the technical points, but the soft skills were missing. They had not been taught or coached, and were also not inherent to her. The unpleasant phlebotomist appeared to me (in my vast, seven minutes' life experience with her) to not be in a good place, either professionally or personally, and I think the unhappiness in one area bled over into the other. Cynthia, my savior, had clearly seen it all. She knew the ways of the world, and she knew what made her fulfilled. While my recollection of her great attention and my subsequent smiling appreciation is not hyperbole, I can more significantly imagine Cynthia smiling more broadly as she left my room. She knew she was good; she knew she did right by me, and she took pride in that. That, right there, I think is indicative of a generational gap. The younger service providers, in general, seem to have less pride in their work. I have seen that professionally—millennials can be less patient to learn a position, do the work well and proudly, and make it their own. A prevailing attitude is that their current stage of life or work is beneath them.

Most caregivers are seriously dedicated, and most realize the impact they can have upon a person—a fellow member of our community—in a potentially dire hour. And maybe that's where I am making more of it than I should—my problems are miniscule compared to some of the other inmates. My point is also wholly reflective of a couple prime points of this narrative:

Atrial Fibrillation is tremendously frustrating, and it can be next-to-impossible to control, let alone understand all of the machinations it and its treatments can take, and how every variable impacts exponentially on the others.

I always strive to be a good customer, a good partner, and, in this case, a good, proactive, and compliant patient. I work very hard to be in decent shape and to follow doctors' orders to avert further arrhythmic complications. I mention that in this section about caregivers because I think it needs to be a two-way street. Several of my caregivers have pointed out that the vast majority (75-80% at any given moment) of my "floormates," are there with easily-preventable problems. Most are diabetic, and many are obese.

And it's only going to get worse. A couple of generations ago, when I was a kid, free time was filled with outdoor play. Even on Minnesota's frozen tundra. We played outside as long as we could. And then we grudgingly trudged indoors…for a home cooked meal. Thank you, Mom and Dad for allowing my brothers and me to play as kids, and run around the neighborhood unattached to electrical cords.

I'm not perfect, but I do what I can to not foist problems on others. If a doctor or a nurse gives me a directive, I will follow it. And therein lies the rub—as my AFib-afflicted brethren understand—there is no clear, consistent remedy for complicated arrhythmics. That's what is frustrating.

———

It is, of course, tougher to define a conversation about good and bad providers when discussing physicians. Most enter the calling realizing it is just that—a call to a particular, highly-demanding (and potentially lucrative) way to serve their fellow man. Most are proud, bordering on arrogant, and I'm okay with that. In fact, I expect that. They've dedicated themselves and consistently performed at a very high level.

The kicker is getting them to relate to a patient, a customer, a human being. The biggest complaint I hear from within and outside the medical industry is that providers to not have enough time, and do not spend enough time with patients. I can understand that is frustrating for them. Almost as frustrating as it is for a patient.

Maybe my complaints about this not-really-life-threatening affliction are just carping on a trifle. I am upright, I am mostly productive, I am able to function within my family and loved ones, and I am not terminal. That ain't so bad.

No, it's not so bad. But it is frustrating. You've heard that word before. You've said that word before. My neighbors have heard that word as Heather and I seem to compete vociferously for the First Vice-President of Frustration position.

"Adam, you can ask 10 different cardiologists (about Atrial Fibrillation in general), and you'll get 11 varying opinions. Add to that baseline all of the variables in your particular case, and it gets only that much more muddied."

Take that statement from a leading cardiologist, in a wealthy, secure suburb in middle America. Then try to imagine any response other than: "so whatinthehell am I supposed to do?!?!?"

The good ones will take time to describe their particular philosophy. That is helpful. It doesn't fix it, but it does help a patient arm himself with more nuggets of knowledge…so that he can advocate for himself.

The real good ones will take all the time you want, and answer your questions—good questions, dumb questions, and questions that seem to be from outer space. My latest round of arrhythmia was often difficult for me to define. Pre-surgery, I could easily identify

Atrial Fibrillation versus Atrial Flutter. And post-surgery I was supposed to be immune from them anyway…but that's another—actually, it is this—story…. But, as I was struggling to define what I was feeling and also define hard trigger points or times, I darn near disqualified one. My first knockout Flutter experience may have been triggered by drinking cold water, post workout. That was a long time ago, and I only noted it then because of the chronology of my morning routine. This latest time around, I thought I was noticing it almost consistently.

It was in a conversation with this "good" provider that I was able to point this out. He responded that yes, incidents can sometimes be vagally-induced. He described it a little further, but we then moved on. We were clearly past trying to pinpoint one smoking gun. After four years, I had buckshot in my blood, and the better question—for me and for the providers—was, what do we do about it?!

In the same paragraph of this conversation, this doctor offered a few ways for me to not trigger episodes. Yes, cold water and other esophageal trauma could be a small trigger. Okay—don't do it.

———

On a bigger scale, I was to exercise in moderation. I thought I had been! And upon this point, I have been gin-clear. I communicate everything. Since this began, I reduced my caffeine intake from superhuman to almost-inhumane. I do have a sweet tooth, but that's part of why I exercise. I do not drink alcohol. We eat well;

balanced meals each night we're home, next-to-no fast food, and a strong aversion to grease when we do indulge. I will enjoy an occasional cigar. No providers have seen fit to curtail any point of my day-to-day-ness.

Until now. He has one point that likely makes sense, and another that has got me flummoxed. An occasional cigar is not going to kill me, but his contention is that I'm too smart for that. There is no tobacco use that is good tobacco use. I probably can't argue with that. He suckered me in by saying I'm too smart....

The other point is the level of exercise. I quantify what I do on a daily and weekly basis. At my peak I would run 22 miles a week, and I was happy doing so. A couple of nurses might have raised half an eyebrow and offered the opinion that: "I wouldn't do much more than that level," but they never instituted an outright prohibition or cap on the trade. As my saga has worn on, I have made a concerted effort to diversify. For one principal reason—I know my joints won't hold up for a lifetime of pavement pounding. Beyond that, I enjoy exercising, and being somewhat in shape, and being able to "play" when I get a chance, and I purely love the hopeful peace of mind that comes from actively preventing future bad health outcomes.

A morning run helps clear my head, and allows me to justify the previous night's dessert. When I run outdoors in the summer it's that much sweeter. When I'm strapped to the treadmill in the basement, well, it makes me really appreciate that outdoor time all the more. It gets me in shape to play tennis (in my mind) like a fifteen-year-old. I may not be a great player, but I love trying to outwork my opponent. Love it.

This physician is a thought-leader in his field. He's published several books on this narrow subject, and on the interrelatedness of overall health. He suggested one of his books to me no fewer than three times.

His earnest suggestion was that I exercise less, and less strenuously. And do yoga.

I have nothing against yoga, in general. I have a few friends who practice it currently, and quite a few more friends who formerly practiced it. One friend spoke glowingly about the concept. He practiced for about three years directly following his divorce. His two favorite distinct memories: yoga pants, and Shavasana. While I don't have a strong stance against either, I am not eager to try to carve out several more hours in my week for a new hobby.

Here's the thing—he might be right. And he might not.

I had a (hard-fought) appointment with my primary EP a couple of days after my dofetilide lock up. I presented my case for prevention, enjoyment, and my fervent dedication to not exceeding my (his) 150 Beats Per Minute heart rate threshold. I make that point very clearly, then and now, because I was amazed at how long my recovery was taking. That is another part of the story, and I will get there…but not now.

My EP's directive du jour was to enjoy exercising for its own sake. And not obsess over the data.

I like the sound of this. It is tough for me to "not obsess over the data," but I will work toward it. My first week after this directive, I ran every morning except the one day a week I have a breakfast meeting. I played tennis two days. That's six days of exercise, and I recorded them all, but I did not track nor worry about my heart rate. It's still been erratic, but I have been feeling better about getting back into my normal life.

And that's been the best diagnosis/directive of late. Maybe that's why he's one of the good ones? I appreciate his release back to normalcy…but the other constant remains—uncertainty. No real diagnosis, no real plan, no tangible improvement or benefit.

At least he communicates, and that is what makes any service provider a standout—from an entry-level desk clerk to a top line cardiologist.

———

I describe my Mayo Clinic experience in more detail elsewhere. Here, though, it rounds out the "Good Provider, Bad Provider" section. The Mayo Clinic is simply the gold standard for modern western medical care. It can probably transcend other industries as well, in relation to customer service and communication.

There may be better technical specialists elsewhere, and particularly on the money-no-object coasts. But overall, the experience trumps, by far, any single effect that one best-ever person could offer. Door-to-door, the level of and expectation to care is unparalleled. Professionalism abounds. And in a kind, thoughtful way.

Nobody is in a hurry. But everything starts exactly smack-dab on time. Despite the reason I was there, I was in heaven.

I'll reinforce an earlier statement that I don't think is controversial. There are spectacular physicians everywhere. And dedicated, technically-proficient nurses, techs and administrators everywhere. Especially in our more metropolitan and moneyed-areas.

But Mayo has got the entire formula. Nordstrom, Mercedes-Benz, Costco, Harvard and Coca-Cola all wrapped up into one.

The Mayo mojo somehow attracts these best and brightest to a Godforsaken southern Minnesota small city. I can call it that because I am a native Minnesotan. And my wife enjoys visiting the state…even when forced to spend eleven days in a Rochester hotel room.

I have a feeling that the Mayo notation on a resume is more significant than just about anything else on a physician's CV. I also assume that indoctrination into the Mayo way can be tough for some of the egoists-turned-doctors. They are terrific ladies and gentlemen from the world over. They're bright and dedicated…and they put their pants on the same way as the rest of us poor people.

As I have mentioned, I try to be a good, educated customer. Part of that goes with not wasting the providers' time. I think they appreciate some preparation, documentation, and maybe even editing of questions beforehand. They didn't rise to the top of their professions to entertain my theories and questions about over-the-counter medications and their television ads.

On my first consultative trip there, I had I think five tests/appointments scheduled. I showed up to my two morning tests on time, and each started right on time. I was 40 minutes *ahead of* schedule right off the bat.

I was of course a little early for my first appointment with a doctor, and checked in nicely at the desk. An aide began taking all of my information and history and preparing me for the doctor's visit. I expected a seven-minute swoop in, a firm declaration, and a treatment directive with little consultation or conversation. I was wrong.

The doctor was kind, affable, and in no hurry. Don't get me wrong—he didn't dawdle, but he spent as much time with us as we needed. He calmly asked a bunch of questions while taking a light physical examination. It was obvious he had internalized the pages upon pages of records I had sent up earlier, but he was more concerned with hearing it directly from me.

In retrospect, I have a feeling he was going through a weeding-out inventory. I am not pooh-pooing anyone's perception about this affliction, but I can imagine that a lot of us get to be whiny and worn out, and then expect a miracle cure without putting in any diligence on our own. I hope I project that I actively work to control what I can. And especially that I do not obliviously aggravate my condition.

I do recall I was nervous going in, like I was really going into an interview. But he put us both at ease. And that is a critical concept—it is absolutely worthless if the patient feels good about a direction, but the spouse is either in the dark, or set against, or feels diminished in opinion. My wife and I communicate differently—but on this topic, we make sure we are on the same page.

Dr. N did not force anything. He gently nudged the conversation, felt out our history, absolutely felt our pain and frustration, and kindly outlined some options. He also did so without disparaging any previous caregivers or their diagnoses and treatments.

I realize this is a little bit contrary to the general theme of the book. The Mayo docs are not omnipotent—obviously, that's why I am writing this months later. Nor certainly do they have a silver bullet that other physicians can't access. But their method, simply by communicating and taking time, goes a great way to making a patient feel good about the future.

The doctors are great, and I think they are afforded the opportunity to function in a system that allows them to be physicians, not manufacturers.

———

After Dr. N referred us to Dr. S, a decision was made, and that's where I stopped being an active patient. We felt great about the decision, and more importantly about the process to get there. And I knew I was okay to quit meddling, advocating and troubleshooting. I was in the right place, and would be back, on my back, in that right place in a few weeks.

———

These doctors had no ego, no loss of face or lifestyle if I chose to go elsewhere or have a different procedure, of even if I ignored it all. They, completely and competently, walked me through the entire scenario, good and bad, and through that process they allowed me to arrive at the "right" conclusion. They fulfilled the first part of their professional obligation. They cannot, and they realize they cannot, force me or sell me on something.

This is a concept that transcends medicine, or, frankly, any industry. The best don't need to be any better than they are, and the certainly do not need to waste breath on forcing a perception.

———

From a practical perspective, who benefits most from this unforced proficiency?

I'm almost a little uneasy drawing this comparison, but Heather and I both felt uneasy in retrospect, in reviewing our consultations with both local surgeons. Both gentlemen were, doubtless, fully capable and wholly respected in their profession and community.

Each was extremely confident that he would be able to handle the procedure, and would give me the best chance for full relief and (almost) no future worry.

They both did a remarkable job at presenting their abilities, capabilities, history and recommendation for my case. What they did not do was examine the data, and the future options in their totality. Neither guy wanted to discuss the pros and cons of other procedures, let alone other non-surgical options.

"Surgeons love to cut." I had a college professor offer that tidbit, and while I'm sure he did not coin the phrase, he sure made it his own. And I love the analogy—especially now. This particular professor was an English professor. He loved the language, he loved all things words, and he loved books. It was his vocation and more so his avocation. He went to great lengths to describe how, because of his affection for the printed page, he worked at it with discipline each and every day. He enjoyed it so much that he worked and worked and honed his craft and opened his eyes and his mind every day to all expressions of the art.

In anything, the more you study, understand, share, the more you appreciate and the higher your core competency. Human nature indicates one's inherent tendency to head to a default, a comfort zone.

When given the chance, surgeons will opt to cut. That was my real takeaway after the local consultations. The more I thought about it, the more I realized the big perspective was missing. In fact, there was no discussion, direct or indirect, about the options of procedures. I'm still not convinced they were even trying to compare apples to apples. I have three different procedures in my notes and research.

These doctors, each independently, saw a "live one" walk into their office, eager for a solution. Damn the options—this is what I do! The more I considered, the more turned off I became.

Peace of mind was the single most substantial takeaway from my consultations and procedures at the Mayo Clinic.

Post-Maze Hospital Release!

AFTER DAYS AND days of tofu smoothies, augmented with three squares a day and not at all burned off by hundreds of laps around my recovery unit's floor, I was ready to resume life. I don't say this critically—they were wholly concerned with my short-term and long-term care…but once I had crossed some threshold, it was time to push me out of the nest. And I was ready, sort of.

My timeline even of the last couple days is a little hazy. I remember I had an Echo, that seemed to take all afternoon. It started with a wheelchair trip to, apparently, Northfield (a nearby city, home to a couple of great colleges that are complete with underground campus passageways—my passage underneath Mayo seemed to go on and on forever). I was tired by the time I got there, and I had to go the bathroom. I'm glad I said something at the time we arrived at the underground nuclear chamber, because once arrived, they were of course ready to hook me up and examine my abdomen from every angle. It took at least 90 minutes. I think I slept during the ride up from the subterranean.

I do not remember them removing the IJ (Intra-Jugular) line, thank goodness. In fact, I am such a wimp that I only vaguely remember being aware of its presence throughout the five or six days it protruded, making me look like a member of the Addams Family. I sort of knew it was there, but I so-vigilantly ignored any confrontation with it, that it was a shock when, during a visit, Heather showed me a photo from earlier in the week. Of course, then it bothered me to no end, until they removed it (which I mercifully do not remember)—that may be why I was so tired for the Echo voyage—I probably had slept even more poorly than usual once I noticed the damn thing.

I do, way too clearly, remember when they removed the wires to my "External Pacemaker." This had been a necessary appliance for a whole bunch of reasons, and by my account, kept me running as I slowly recovered and my naturally-slow heart grudgingly began to work normally.

The "Pacer," as they called it was like a huge remote control. But not wireless. It was loosely attached to me by two thin wires, which were somehow loosely placed within my heart's protective sac. They led out of small, non-sutured and unsecured holes in the middle of my abdomen. I do *not* know how everything stayed in-place and plugged-in. And I did *not* examine closely. The external Pacer was able, proximately, to send an electrical signal that would trigger beats. The machine did keep me running, and also caused some consternation (and amusement?) among the medical staff.

As the tech came in to remove this, what may have been my final encumbrance, he tried to describe to me what I should be prepared for: "It will feel like, well, two thin wires being pulled out." "It won't hurt, but you will know it is happening."

That was an accurate description, and the first wire's removal, while vaguely discomforting, was not at all painful. The second started similarly…until I felt a flood of warmth running down my side, past my hip, and almost immediately pooling by my hip. The tech was nice enough to keep pulling (and pulling, and pulling, it seemed—the thing must have been three feet long), so there was no pause in the action. All was complete, and he quickly swooped in and mopped up on my chest. I knew myself well enough to not look closely. But as I got up to head into the bathroom and do some more active cleaning, I did glance down at the pool of bright red blood on the stark white sheets. My takeaways were: boy, I'm glad I did not look at that at the time, and wow—that really is bright red—that must be a good sign!

I believe that particular bloodletting occurred near the end of my penultimate day on campus. Heather had planned to stay with me through dinner and we'd watch some TV for a few hours. The theory was that, as I was becoming more and more lucid each day, we might like to spend some time together. As I think back now, I was not very lucid at all.

Apparently I was in and out of sleep and not very pleasant company at all. Go figure. I was mostly half-asleep, until she wanted to change the channel from whatever awful show I was insistent upon watching. At that point, many times over, I would wake up, maintain that I was indeed paying attention, and she should quit trying to pull a fast one on me. I was a peach. But she was wonderfully patient to the not-wonderful patient.

I mention this story because it still boggles my mind how "out of it" I was then, and would continue to be even for several weeks while at home.

My real check out took much of the next day. Trips to the Pharmacy, conferences and approvals from reams of medical professionals…and then a quick signature. Heather ran back to the hotel and graciously retrieved the car, and I had one final wheelchair ride downstairs to wait by the front door.

I shoehorned myself into the large SUV—it is amazing, how, after being coddled for a week, what a challenge even simple real-world moves can be—and we went back to Heather's home away from home. It was a fine hotel…but after 11 days, Heather was ready to scream when she walked in the lobby (she'd only done it a dozen times a day, at least…). I think I changed clothes, and we went out for a light dinner.

Following the logic that while traumatized, a patient may not enjoy food at the time nor ever again in the future, I was not crazy about a big sit-down dinner, but Heather certainly deserved one. The problem was that I could not drive and thereby allow her to enjoy a well-deserved flagon of good wine. It turns out she was not very hungry either, but we did go to a restaurant we'd been to a few times already, and had enjoyed. To keep it light, we each had a small salad and an appetizer order of gnocchi. Both plates were disappointingly salty, and we only picked at them. It was too bad because we had been looking forward to a nice meal "on the outside."

Dinner past us, though, we moved on to more important things! Ice cream. She had kindly already scoped out the Dairy Queen's location, and was more than happy to take me for my first post-surgery Blizzard. What a saint!

It was thick and frozen enough to get back to the hotel, where I sluggishly attempted to shovel it into my tiny mouth. Heather took a shower to wash off the hospital grunge, and I sank into the couch. I made good, but slow progress…until I began to wear said Blizzard. I clearly remember the first missed spoonful. It was in slow motion (everything I did was in slow motion), and even slower as I tried to spoon it off my sloping, non-muscular chest. I wandered into the bathroom to thank her again, and let her laugh at me. And she did. And she took pictures, which she happily sent to friends and family. Adam was free, and he was enjoying ice cream! He could not feed himself cleanly, but he was sure enjoying it. The tougher part was that as I tried to finish the damned thing, it became tougher and tougher to find my mouth. No matter how hard I concentrated, it became slipperier and slipperier. But I was free, and thrilled to be in a lousy hotel bed, feeling really lousy myself, but with my wife by my side.

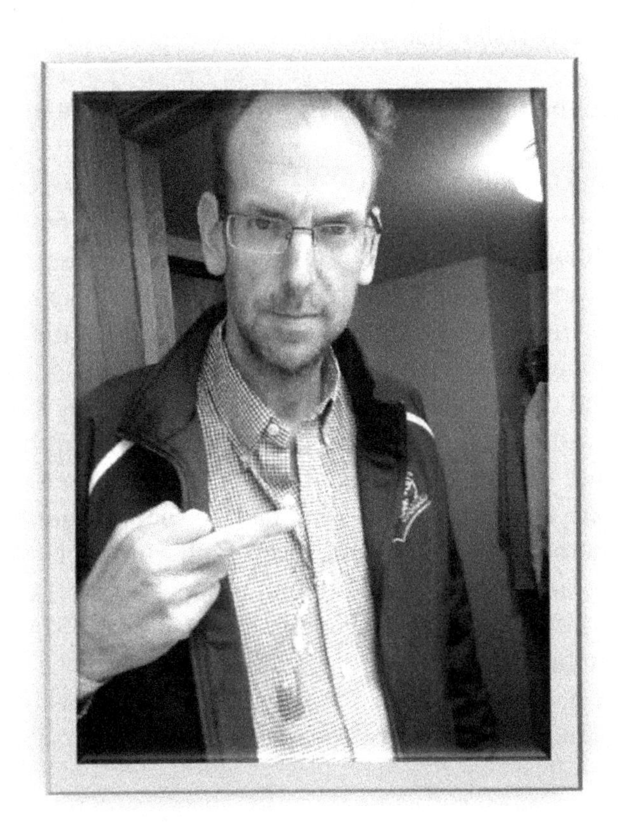

I know I did not sleep well, but she never complained (that I can recall, anyway), and we were eager to rest, make the trip home, and rest some more.

Even without sleeping much, I still awoke early. Way too early for good marital communication, so I stayed quiet. In general, when we take a road trip, I am eager to get moving. I will still often get up and go through my normal morning routine, while not-patiently waiting. I do know enough to not hover—she somehow does not move any faster that way.

But on this, the first day of the rest of my life, I was patient. She needed to sleep and I was barely smart enough to realize that. My exercise in patience was even more vigorous because of the fact that I could do absolutely nothing to help. I barely dressed myself, and then tried to read. I had brought plenty of books to kill my sitting-around time, but I read very little and comprehended even less. The morning minutes ticked by, and Heather began doing everything to get us loaded and ready to go. She may have been a little frustrated because we did, of course, bring a lot of stuff—not that I needed anything. But she had to be prepared for Minnesota weather, and we both brought work stuff…and then my dad brought a bunch of stuff down from his house in Minneapolis. It was nice of him to "clean out," but it was maybe tough timing. Especially as we had to keep some room for our 65# dog, who was undoubtedly going to be pretty excited to see us, eventually.

We got all the loot and laundry loaded, and were almost ready to go. I have no idea what time it was, but I knew that the sun was overhead, and it was now warm. On our way out of town, we had to stop for sustenance. We stopped by our other favorite place in town, a Whole

Foods-style co-op. Heather wanted a fancy coffee and a muffin, and she declared that I needed a smoothie.

Don't tell the ASPCA:

If I had four legs, my lovely wife would be in jail.

It was already an abnormally warm Minnesota day, but per habit, I was wearing a button-down (always, in recovery!) shirt, and flannel at that. I am well-conditioned to always be cold. I even had a warm-up jacket handy, for the inevitable temperature debate during the trip home. But I had never counted on being too warm.

As I was clearly incapacitated, Heather assumed I could not be trusted with the car keys. Maybe she was right, but I was sweating. Her quick trip inside seemed to take hours. On a normal August day, I would open the door, enjoy the breeze, and maybe even walk around a little. On this lovely day, though, there was a jackhammer working on the parking lot...approximately three feet from my right ear. I could do nothing except sweat and be patient. My two favorite things.

———

I think I was pleasant once my savior returned, as we were able to laugh about it…for the next six or so hours. I enjoyed my smoothie, a few sips of Heather's coffee, and a scone or two as we settled in for a nice trip.

My grumblings aside, she was an excellent captain. I was glad that we had driven. Flying would have been an all-day affair in its own right, and exceedingly more complicated, to boot. Our trip was pretty smooth. We made it to the wonderful folks who had taken care of Moxie, just before rush hour. I had been concerned about this timing, as once we picked her up, we then had to cross the entire north-south metropolitan area, but she had it down.

We pulled into our garage at 5:00. The heavens opened up at 5:06, and I was safely already ensconced in the living room watching the storm.

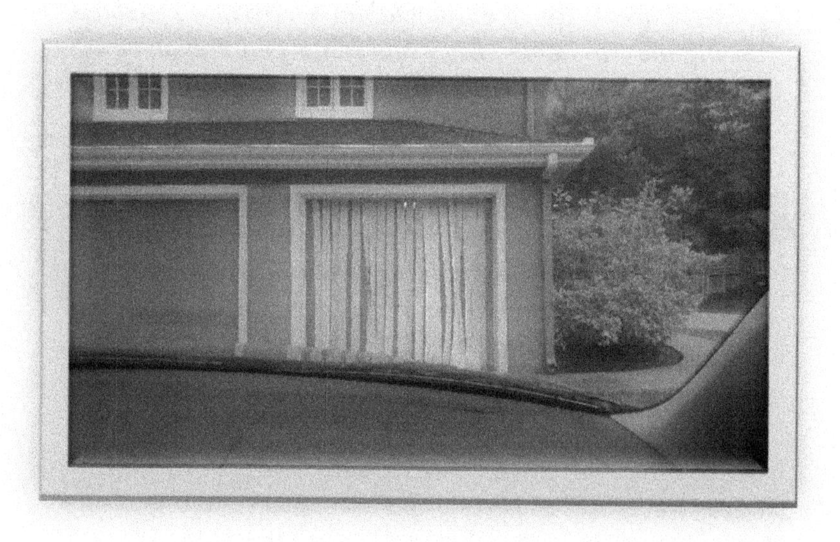

Our dear friends and neighbors had a great meal ready for us, and everyone enjoyed a hearty laugh at how the kids had decorated the garage to welcome us home. It was a great feeling to be home.

Even though I was not in my right mind, because my body was miserable, it was warmingly pleasant to be there and to sit with the dog, as Heather raced around putting things in order—which is really what makes her feel good!

It was great to be home.

(Self)-Recuperation

IT WAS GREAT to be home. Especially because that meant I could start getting stronger. Right away!

I could start eating like a normal person, and I soon could start exercising as I'd like. I was soon going to be better than ever, and things were to be great. I couldn't wait. I had a couple of nice coloring-book-style notebooks describing how I was to stretch, and of course use my quickly-becoming-hated inspirational respirometer. It was all there in black and white—my road to recuperation and strength and longevity was before my very eyes. This, combined with my personal history and knowledge base would serve me well.

I don't totally mean to mock the instructional manual. While the illustrations were fairly facile, it was still helpful to see for the sake of proper form. That was principally what I was seeking—especially as my body had been stressed in unnatural and unprecedented ways. If the book showed I was supposed to hold a yardstick or a golf club and stretch over my head in that manner, so be it—that's what I would do…over and over and over.

And there comes one strong word of caution. Do not overdo it. I'll combine that with the other critical concept: stay on your pain medication, and stay ahead of the pain. The final word here: again, *do not overdo it.* In any capacity. It's easy to do an extra five sets of arm stretches while watching *Dragnet* reruns for the fifth day of the week…but there is a reason the book says to do only three. Especially on your first week home.

For that first week I did stay on my pain meds. Alternating acetaminophen and oxycodone, I could, at least in hopeful theory, feel my brain coming back to life. It is still boggling how foggy I had been, and how long it took to clear out. My medical directions were even hazy, but I roughly recall: breathe. Breathe a lot, do the exercises in the book, and begin walking as I was able.

Sure, easy enough. And I was optimistic. Way too optimistic, and even more so than my lovely wife had hoped.

Heather went back to work that first week, although she did spend a couple days working from home just to wean me off hour-by-hour supervision. I was okay, and quickly moved into a routine. I would get up and do my stretching and breathing, and write them down in a little notebook. I would then have breakfast (keep eating, dummy!), sit down and watch some TV, and then take a little nap. I'd repeat that in the afternoon, but with a sweet snack taking the place of eggs or breakfast cereal.

Life was pretty good, despite how miserable I felt mentally and physically. I don't offer emotionally, because my brain still felt pickled, and did not allow for feelings to register. I was clearly hamstrung mentally.

So slow, mentally, that I did not register enough to balk when Friday evening rolled around, and Heather suggested a somewhat-normal routine. Sure, I'd be happy to stand outside and grill dinner. As I first walked out, I did have the wherewithal to point out that I could not/should not stretch my arms chest and shoulders so much as to uncover the grill. Heather broke free of the indoor chores and helped me with that.

And I stood there, growing more miserable by the second. This was way above my cleared-for-activity-level. But I didn't want to rain on her parade. She of course, deserved a good meal, at home—where we had been longing to be, together. But as my head drooped during dinner, we both realized it had been too much too soon.

My first week was intentionally weak. I took my time, and hobbled around the house in a daze, literally trying to remember how to breathe. I then planned a meteoric rise for the next week. I began walking. Slowly, of course. I did it in the morning, when my strength was at its zenith. One quarter of a mile the first day, and all the way up to a half mile by Friday. And halfway in I got overconfident. Wednesday or Thursday I quit my prescription painkillers. I was okay for a day or two, and then was precipitously worse, the escalating pain staying with me for at least a week.

The daily pain began as a dull ache everywhere. I figured that was normal and I could live with it. But the chest pain was acute, and growing.

I was still oversensitive, and overprotective of my sternum. That is part of the reason the several specific stretching exercises are prescribed—to prevent the protective "hunching" of shoulders, back and neck. But I may have overdone that stretching—it was tight when I was doing it, but that meant it was working, right? But by the late afternoon…and the middle of the night, the sharp, biting pain through my chest, shoulders, back and neck was crippling.

I'm still not mastering the language to describe it. I know many have been through significantly more traumatic events, but this was excruciating. Each breath, shallow even as they were, was excruciating. For several days I kept with my routine, but I did so without sleeping. I was miserable through the day, and worse through the night. There was no way to lie down comfortably. Not, anyway, if I wanted to breathe at the same time.

I had no way to be comfortable, either vertically or horizontally. In an attempt to mitigate the collateral damage, I moved to a guest room for a couple of nights (after trying to start the night in our bedroom, as normal). Basically, I would walk across the hall, crawl into that bed, sweat all over it, and finally sink to an hour or two of sleep before Heather woke up in the morning. As she was up and not disturb-able any more, I moved back to the master bedroom…where I spouted more pain-sweat for an hour or two before actually getting up as Heather headed out the door for work.

I spent several days actively, and yet tentatively, tapping the length of my clavicle—I was entirely convinced that I had somehow broken it, and that's what was leading to the searing pain with each shallow breath.

Several frantic calls to Rochester, Minnesota basically came down to one concept—you're not going to be magically repaired this quickly, you've gone through major trauma, and you should make sure to use the proper pain medications!

There are no valor medals for being strong enough to kick the narcotics early. General comfort aside, when one's body expends a great deal of energy suffering from the pain, the body cannot spend what energy it has toward repairing itself. That, and the universal fact that sleep is tremendously therapeutic. Dummy.

I resumed the narcotics, and while initial dulling of the pain was pretty quick, it still took a couple days to get fully into my system and provide sustainable relief.

One word of caution—plan ahead! When I had my one post-surgery look-see one week after I had been home, I had high hopes of killing my painkillers soon. When I was given the "gee, everything looks okay" prognosis (which was really only that the wounds were healing, and were not showing signs of infection), I of course became overconfident. A couple days after that is when I did quit the oxycodone—which was really a very small amount—40 mg. over the course of a full day, at its maximum—but those 5-10 mg. every six hours had really built up a protective barrier.

Because I felt okay, and the nurse and doctor thought I was progressing fine, I did not request an extended prescription. If, worse came to worse and I wanted to continue them, I figured one quick call to Mayo and we could then pick them up at my corner pharmacy an hour later. Wrong. As Opioids are, appropriately so, heavily controlled, a provider cannot prescribe, or even extend a prescription remotely. They need to physically lay eyes upon you.

After I learned my lesson and began a strict regimen, I started counting the pills. And I had to make another trip back to my local doctor before they would extend it, and that extension was absolutely medically necessary—no two ways about that.

———

Once back into an intelligent pain management regimen, my strength curve did turn skyward. Within two weeks I was walking a total of five miles a day. And that's when I began to get (more) restless, and eager for professional rehabilitation advice.

———

I realize a lot of my carping about pain and discomfort and slow recuperation may sound trite…but again, I was fortunately, a healthy, vigorous forty-some-year-old, who had never previously been incapacitated. It was tough. As I consider in arrears, I'm not sure I would put myself through it again. But as I consider more, I do reinforce my initial logic—this surgery gave me the best chance at a long-term fix. Even that chance was worth the recovery misery.

Before I get to the details with the "professionals," I have two bits of layman's advice for recovery.

Technology can be your friend. I had begun using a GPS watch several years ago as my one nod to technology when running. I do like to track my progress, and I really also like being able to plan and explore different routes by always knowing my exact distance. While I had a good knowledge of all variations on a three-mile loop through my neighborhood, I did not have a grasp on smaller increments. As I began hobbling around in my recovery, it was a great and simple tool to help me track my progress in those miniscule increments. Even for peace of mind, I highly recommend it as a useful tool.

Friends can also be your friend. While I made exactly zero friends while in my professional rehab routine, I did enjoy even a very little companionship while wandering. Some friends made very considerate offers to join me, but I was really not feeling social. Where I did enjoy some interaction was when I began to make early-morning trips and saw some old neighbors in familiar routines. I had not advertised my procedure, but it was nice as loose acquaintances inquired and were genuinely curious and hopeful for me. And when I needed further interaction, I could go around and deliver the mis-delivered mail that landed in my mailbox.

The corollary to this is that I passed a lot of happy dog walkers. While Moxie the Doberman was the best recovery companion a guy could ever hope for, she was beside herself not understanding why I was not taking my walks *with her!* Dobermans are known as "Velcro dogs," and she is no exception. She was lockstep with each stumble within the house, while using her eyes to implore to me that she wanted to walk *with me, outside!* She did not seem to understand the squirrel-chasing and sternum-ripping potential paradox.

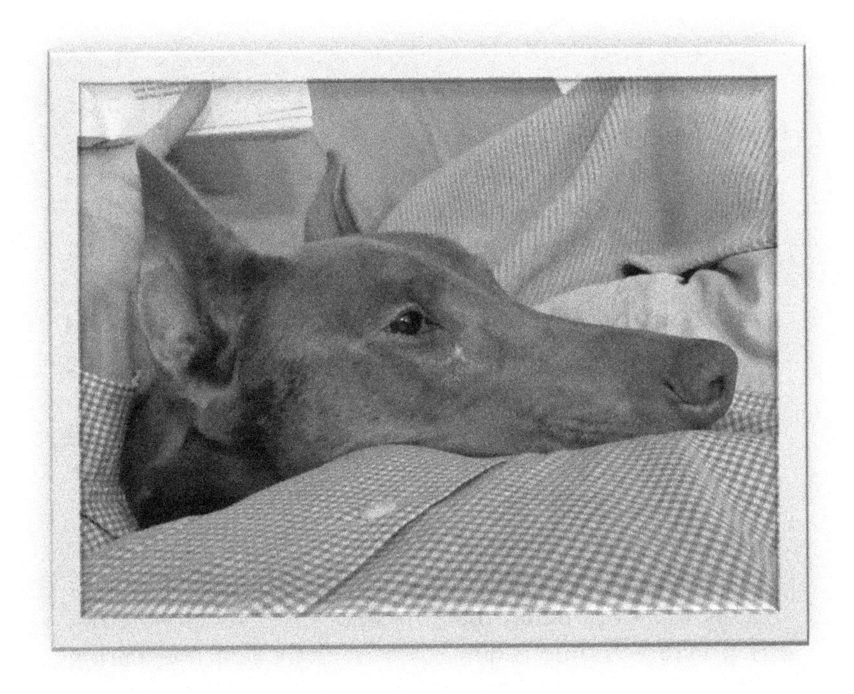

Cardiac Rehabilitation

UPON MY DISCHARGE from Mayo I had a nice, and lukewarm precis to the concept of official, hospital-style rehabilitation. The most significant takeaway was that it might be worth considering…if—and only if—insurance would cover it.

Their fervent reinforcement of this concept should have told me all I needed. But I was dedicated to taking all the proper steps toward my rehabilitation. I had decided that I would do it right, and would follow all providers' orders, going in to the surgical commitment. And especially on the other side.

And why wouldn't I? This was a new beginning! This was even better than my original ASD closure fix. I'd take the time, under care of dedicated and caring professionals, and they would be able to guide me though the sternum-strengthening journey. I would get out of my running routine, and use this as an opportunity to cross-train more.

Unfortunately, I was also still stoned upon my release from Mayo, and I was unable to read the indelible ink between the lines of the insurance caveat regarding outpatient rehab.

———

I am glad I tried it, at the very least so that I can now bitch about it. But it was a colossal waste of time, and a special strain of psychological angst.

To start with, my local hospital was going through a computer system transition, and they could not return a phone call, answer questions, or God forbid, schedule anything to save their lives...or, maybe more aptly, to continue mine.

So, when I finally got a call back, I was at four weeks out from surgery. And fairly into my own routine. Walking was my best therapy, and stretching was equally important. I had done those diligently. Perhaps even over-zealously, and that was part of my attraction to "supervised" rehab. It is entirely possible for one to overdo it, even in simple stretching and strolling. And I did, a few times even in that first month home. I was back to work on a truncated schedule, but was eager to work in a work out, three times a week (I would still do my home routine the other days).

———

I need to offer that not all associated with the program are evil. Just the majority. They generally had a one-size-fits-all, government-style-sense-of-job-security, and feeling that they were well entrenched in the system. Most. Not all. But the weak ones would come around soon, I was sure.

The first call I got was to ask me to come for an evaluation/orientation. Great! But what took so long? "Well, they actually recommend you don't start cardiac rehab until at least five weeks post-surgery." Fine—that may be the case, but my cardiologist's office should have clarified that as I had been calling. Or someone should have called me back to mention that.

Anyway, the young lady that did call me was very diligent. She was glad that my surgery was covered for rehab, and pointed out that often valve jobs and some bypasses are not covered. She was so diligent that she showed me her notes that she called and received pre-approval *twice!*

After five minutes' worth of paperwork, I then headed into a cramped conference room for orientation. Even in my drastically weakened state, I've never felt so alive as when I looked around that room for comparison. Yes, most were typical cardiac patients; older than me and larger than me. In retrospect, I am very glad for their sake that cardiac rehab exists—there is a real need and many of these patients needed guidance for that first step, and second step, etc.

That first session (orientation) took about fifteen minutes. It should have taken seven. This particular "Exercise Specialist" studied under the repetition model of communication. If, in her mind, something was important, she said it twice. That was everything. It was frustrating. It was frustrating.

I really did have empathy for my fellow inmates. We were all weak, worn out, wrung out (having been through the ringer) and probably scared. I now retrospectively recognize that I was a little frightened, in the back of my head. I also know I did not acknowledge it then. I was eager to get moving, and began growing impatient with that first meeting.

I recognize that the nurses, administrators, and "Exercise Specialists" were trying to play to the center of their audience. And I was clearly and proudly an outlier. But I was never a jerk about it, no matter how poor their memories were nor how inapplicable to me a session or topic.

My first "session" was an overview. We did not do anything rehabilitative, but you can bet Obama's bottom dollar that insurers were billed for it as a full session. We were given nametags, taught how to weigh ourselves (and write it down—after shouting it out across the room for the nurses to record), take our heart rate (using counting, and multiplication!), and then finally how to hook up our occasionally-sanitized monitors.

I was given a nice postcard with session times listed, and sort of asked when I wanted to be there. It was not a requirement to pre-register, or even to come to the same session per day and week, but it was sort of requested. Like a lot of sort-of-rules there. I explained that my schedule was going to need to be fairly flexible—I was just getting back into work, and needed to find varying times through the week that might fit.

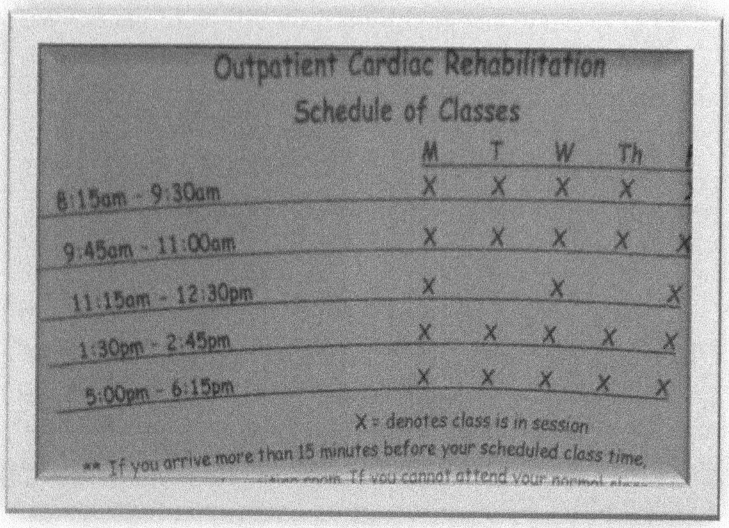

Maybe I set myself up for failure by not rooting down in one particular session. Part of that was my schedule, and part of that was my trying to find a less-annoying session. I know I can be irritable when I don't feel good, or am tired, or am "forced" to do something I don't enjoy, or am not as proficient at something as I'd like. With Cardiac Rehabilitation, I was all of the above. I still maintain, though, that I slapped on my pod face every day, smiled, and went through my routine with near-zero editorializing.

Much like my own imposed programs post-arrhythmia and post-procedure, I did start slow, but was soon eager to push myself. Especially now, in the main lodge of the Johnson County Buick Owners' Club.

I'm not sure which were worse—the inmates or the wardens. I survived by trying to not care, but I do feel bad for the patients for whom this is a literal lifeline. They are clinging to life-saving guidance from inattentive personnel, and they often don't have the tools to do this on their own or the resources to seek other avenues. And they can't quit, or self- graduate.

I won't harp on the patients, but it is a great example of a few ruining the good by not having any adhered-to rules. I'm not talking about any risky or life-threatening behavior, but it was not a professional setting—and that comes from those collecting a paycheck.

There was the guy who set his shoes on a desk at the beginning and end of each session. He was one clearly there for the social outlet. I really can't fault him for that, but the staff didn't care to hold him to any standards of decorum as he bothered the others. I'm fairly tough—I can handle it. I didn't like listening to his stupid or offensive jokes, but I think he learned to not bother me early on. The others, who were not quite out of earshot as he caught up with his buddies, were not so lucky.

There was the guy who took a leak every day and never washed his hands. Silently, I thanked him for ramping up my already borderline-maniacal sanitization routine. By code, I am sure, the room was well-equipped with hand sanitizer foam and wipe stations throughout. But nobody used them. For my first day or two I felt a little prissy about wiping down each machine *before* I used it. Decorum suggests one do so afterwards, but after taking stock of the status quo, I quickly strengthened my internal code and pride, and did what I knew was right—especially what was right for me.

It's next to impossible to cross that guy-code line of browbeating a stranger into proper personal hygiene. With that, I was floored that the women "running" the program never preached sanitization—either from a simple issue of human decency, or God forbid because it's a bad practice to spread germs within a hospital while vulnerable people are at their *most* vulnerable!

We were at the beginning of a political season, and while we all have opinions, I do not think it is one's naturalized right or obligation to share them with everyone in the room. These were not the Lincoln-Douglas debates. These were more along the lines of, at their most basic: "Anyone who would like that guy is a moron." "Oh, you don't agree—well, there we are, you're a moron." It's tough to argue with logic like that, and I was not going to try. It may be a universal law of humanity, but the more closed-minded some of these guys were, the more open-mouthed they were. Some of the sessions primarily populated with these primates were principally puerile in nature. Or more accurately, as puerile as a handful of 70-year-old get-out-of-the-house-ers can be.

Another constituency was a group of enthusiastic, social, fast-walking (and fast-talking) ladies. They were mostly harmless, and I can't complain about them. It was an interesting social observation, though, throughout. This group had a core that was maintained while I was ensconced near-endlessly. One or two satellite biddies would "graduate," and new birds would cycle in. The real interesting part was watching the previously quiet ladies then move up a step in the grandchild-brag pageant.

Sort of interesting to watch, and often fairly sad at the same time. Exacerbated by the staff's "throw them to the wolves" lack of consideration.

And at the far end of the spectrum is the person who really, really needs to be there. They're moving slowly, they're often dropped off by a spouse (who may be waiting nervously in the waiting room), and they mostly had a hollow look in their eyes. It is a frightening thought; it was sad to see. Recalling it helps me maintain a modicum of perspective. I was not there after a heart attack, a stroke, or an emergency bypass. I had had time to prepare, I had decades ahead of me, and hopefully those were to be strong decades. Most of these customers were reconciling how to hang on, and maintain a life, while severely altering their lifestyle. When possible, I would extend myself to orient them even a little bit. The simple act of knowing how to turn on an exercise machine could be daunting.

I do not say that capriciously or caustically. It was tough to watch. There were plenty of things (and many things to this day, exercise or otherwise) that I need repeated before I catch on. When these patients came in to an unknown environment, surrounded by people who all knew what they were doing, it may have seemed insurmountable.

One simple element to help these people assimilate would to treat them like valued customers. A better point would be to treat these people like human beings. Maybe an introduction to another newbie, or a buddy system, or even a one- or two-day handholding would help a lot of these people be more comfortable. The current system of "put on your nametag, and shout your weight and how you're feeling today" was not a model of a caring system.

In case you cannot yet discern, I seem to have the strongest opinions about the "care" givers and administrators of the cardiac rehabilitation program at my local hospital.

While I was not on heavy painkillers anymore once I started rehab, it was fairly clear that I was not totally clear. Perhaps that allowed me to act like an automaton early on, and not push back as much as I would were I functioning normally. As that fog began to lift, I paid more attention to the operation. Perhaps boredom, perhaps trying to troubleshoot it, perhaps just trying to identify if it was all in my head.

What I could discern was that there was no one in charge. Nor was there any continuity, day to day. The only hierarchy in the "Lord of the Flies" management model was based upon volume. And I don't mean volume of customers served. I mean simple vociferousness. And I might mean a thinly-veiled reference to the "Piggy" character.

The work did get done, and each session ran to full completion, more or less—although never on time (especially the one session each day right after lunch!). That was one point of frustration. A primary frustration was seeing the patients in real need struggle aimlessly or uncomfortably. When Piggy might catch on that help was needed, her primary method was to shriek across the room before waddling across it for an appropriate, private but still room-reverberatingly-loud conversation.

Again, my concerns are petty. I realize that. But simply expecting professionalism should not be outside the bounds. Especially in a medical situation, when patients are at a significant turning point in their lives.

I do also realize that these bad-sorority-house harridans probably do play well to a portion of the crowd. Some of the gentlemen were happy to hang around young women—especially young women of their similar level of physical fitness. And I'm sure some of the grandmotherly-types enjoyed sharing grandchildren stories. From what I could unfortunately gather, the more details about diapers and upset stomachs the better!

Back to the "management" analysis. What little rhyme or reason there was to the system kept eluding me. For two weeks I thought I was in fat city, so to speak—I had anticipated Piggy's off day, and made that the cornerstone of my week. By the third week, no avail—

the system got the better of me and I was back balancing my physical well-being against my psychological strain.

Beyond that, though, no hierarchy or accountability. Adding credence to my observations were incidents of eye-rolling by some of the more responsive or perceptive staffers. One nice RN whispered to me, away from prying eyes "Wow—I bet you're really looking forward to being finished here."

To that, I believe the RNs cycle down into the purgatory of rehab from their normal hospital duties—generally on the cardiac floor. They were invariably the most professional ones, and also the ones with zero vested interest in professionalizing the room.

———

Each session began with stretching. Totally appropriate and necessary. What was not appropriate was how we were described to stretch. One of the vaunted Exercise Specialists would take a seat (yes, she'd sit down to stretch) at the front of the room, and we sheep would gather in a somewhat-semicircle. She'd then begin waving her arms, describing how we should move if, in fact, we could move our arms in a reasonable fashion. We'd then move to legs, hips, lower body and the like. She would describe how we should touch our toes, if, in fact one was able to do so.

My statement here is less an indictment of careless medical care, and more of our cumbersome business climate. In order to have a particular job, one should be able to do that particular job. If a young, seemingly otherwise healthy woman is grossly overweight, or obese, she cannot do the job of "Exercise Specialist!" And I should not be subjected to watching her not try to do that particular job.

I know—I'm not their core constituent. Most of their audience (because it was often a show—shitshow or otherwise) probably was comfortable sharing those challenges and not being trained by Charles Atlas.

The stretching is the best example. Especially because I am not very flexible. As my years pass, though, I make a more concerted effort to stretch before exercising. It allows me to be more effective, in less pain afterwards, to be able to do more and for longer (in both minutes and years), and also stave off injury.

But I never *learned* anything in these sessions. And more unfortunately, the people that really needed to increase flexibility and muscle tone learned even less.

As Piggy would tell us to touch her toes, there was no toe-touching tutelage. Even as I, a stiff, well, not-quite-stiff, work to stretch, I do not totally touch my toes. But I do understand the concept, and concentrate on actually stretching the muscles—feeling it in my hamstrings and calves. By Piggy's example, touching our toes consisted of bending one's leg (from her seated position), and grabbing the cuff of her scrubs in order to hold her ankle in suspension. That is not a good example, and becomes even more glaring with the absolute lack of description of the process or its goal.

———

For me, it reinforced my motivation. We all have our challenges. I renewed the pledge to myself that I will do everything I can to make my doctors' lives easier, for the balance of mine.

I also continually pledge to always put my best foot forward in anything I try. I am not a perfect human being, but I do my best to show up, be prepared, and never short myself on effort.

When one is physically incapable of doing a job, it is frustrating. When she does not put in the effort, it makes it worse. And yes, I wrote "she." Every employee in the Cardiac Rehabilitation unit was female. Strange.

———

Sex Does Not Sell

"Let's talk about sex, baby!" I knew it the minute I heard the squawkingly-butchered version of that mid-nineties bubblegum-rap anthem. I should have turned around and walked back out the door. I was only four steps into the room, but was unfortunately directly adjacent to the nurses' nest, from where this awful concept was being cawed by an awful voice. I wondered how they were going to measure the pressure of my blood when said substance had curdled at that very moment.

I flinched, but I kept going. I must have been in an overly-benevolent mood that morning, because I remember specifically trying to not make a scene. But the concept was absolutely cringe-worthy. It was Piggy, in near-full voice. Titillating the masses of oversized asses, and nearly causing my entryway whiplash.

I am happily in the minority. I was not a rapt student during the nutrition lecture telling us how to eat heart-healthy, to avoid heart attacks. I did sit patiently when they tried to share tips to help us create exercise habits and patterns. And I was polite when afterwards, I asked if moving forward I might skip some of these symposia, and continue exercising, as I was a different case.

And yes, I kept my lips zipped even through a dubious opening. But, as is typical, none of the other nurses in the room sought to muzzle our performer. And therefore she was encouraged to continue and increase in volume...and the others eagerly followed suit.

Piggy jiggled around the pre-session paperwork and registration time shrieking "I'm doing our lecture today, we're all going to talk about sex!"

Head down, Adam, eyes averted. Hang in there. Keep cool.

I think I've done a pretty good job of not blowing my top. Not even when she complained that there was no movie like "Debbie Does Dallas" that corresponded to her first name. Nor when she swooned and moaned and speculated about a particularly dreamy doctor (that I happen to know well. You're welcome, Doc, that I have not tortured you with this knowledge).

So I had zero hopes that handing her this megaphone was going to lead to a professional, useful conversation. No way, no how, and certainly no way based upon the entryway serenade.

Following her lead, about 30% of the group was on board the boat. The rest of us were varying levels of uncomfortable. A few of the enthusiasts had been clearly waiting for this opportunity, as it was not the kind of conversation you have around the dinner table, or at work, or with a church group…or anywhere! The principal foil for Piggy was a retired junior-college professorial type, whose career had apparently revolved around the romantic lives and according anatomical anomalies of various types of rhinoceros.

I kept it zipped (my mouth, and everything else), and tried to stay within my arbitrary exercise level limits. I toughed out the session, and made it clear that I was not going to stick around for the lecture. My check-out procedure was hindered by bureaucracy and lack of attention by the other clerks. And after 75 minutes overall, my blood had boiled up through my eyeballs.

I did not swear it off then and there, but as the day wore on, I had a moment of significant clarity. It was not worth my time, my insurer's money, and certainly not worth the strain on my psyche.

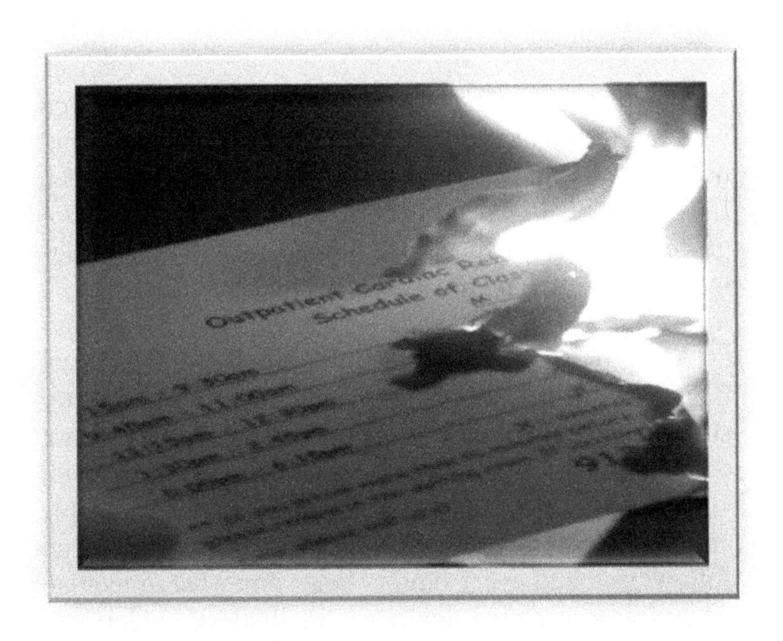

In conclusion, the "structured" rehabilitation program was a bad fit for me. With no cohesive management, there was no continuum of care for each patient. I cannot tell you how many times I had the same conversation—all at my behest—with several different personnel. I was routinely trying to reeducate them on my history, procedure, and goals. And they all had a blank look on their faces as they mentally lumped me in with the heart disease patients. Frustrating for me, and more concerning, the real heart disease patients—who could really benefit from a caring hand—were turned into faceless cattle.

Piggy runs the community, and the hospital has an apparently untended but tidy profit center.

—

Now many months in to post-surgery recovery, I am working to broaden my perspective. I realize that I am not a fitness or nutrition guru. But I am stubborn. When I set a personal goal, I will hit it. I am not a natural or graceful runner, but each painful pavement pound brings me daily improvement. That's what keeps me going.

And so when I began my mid-thirties' physical improvement in earnest—to make sure I was in better shape at 40 than at 20, I did it. Through stubborn dedication. I did not read a bunch of books or consult with a nutritionist. I exercised more and ate less. Simple enough for me to remember each and every day, and follow each and every day. I was somewhat draconian when left to my own devices—small snack, yogurt and protein shakes for lunch three or four days a week. If I had a business lunch, it was a salad.

I felt great. Yes, aches and pains on my joints were pretty regular, but I began to feel like I was getting back to my ideal body type. Even at 6'2', I am not meant to carry 200#. And as I ate less during the day, I felt better through the days, morning noon and night. When I would have a normal American's lunch, I was sluggish in the afternoon, and often even into the next day.

That is part of what is frustrating now. Through the first several months of my recovery, friends and family were imploring me to EAT MORE!

I never had an appetite problem, but that may have been the perception. Even my first month or two after surgery, people were coming out of the woodwork to tell me how much better I looked. For many months prior, I had been too skinny. I thought that since I felt better, I looked better. Not accurate.

Post-surgery, I ate frequently—generally still as well as we do normally, but I indulged the "pack on some pounds" concept. Dairy Queen here we come! Thank you, Heather, for driving me there…dozens of times.

And as I filled out a little (not muscle of course, mind you) the commenters' common refrain was that my color was great. That sure made me feel good to hear that…but I also began to connect the dots. It was entirely possible that I had overdone it for the past several years. While I had never been "sick," I now fully believe that over-exercise contributed to that unhealthy pallor. And while I'm still convinced that for me, morning exertion adds energy throughout the day, while I had been in this compromised state of un-circulation for a couple years, I was doing myself more harm than good.

———

As I had been impatient getting back to fighting shape, I was trying to look at the bigger picture.

One of the (actual good) nurses at cardiac rehab exclaimed happily at weigh-in: *"You've lost weight—great!"* Except that I was not trying to lose any weight. She was sincere in her praise, as she was simply programmed to counsel every single patient through that door that a primary goal toward cardiac health is to lose weight. *"Look at me, lady—I look like something grown in a dark closet. Withering away further will not be good. I am trying to gain weight. It's right there as a primary goal on my chart."*

The lesson I did take was the only thing that dovetailed with my stated goal going into rehab—I wanted to learn how to exercise differently, and *more effectively, long-term.*

I began to enjoy the elliptical machine as a cardio-intensive alternative to running which was not an option now anyway. I also began to enjoy the feeling of light weight work (despite being reminiscent of high school ski-training torture).

My attraction to the weight work was to regain what little muscle I had had in my upper body before that bloody July day. I had never been described as muscular, but my pre-run stretching regimen did include daily push-ups and sit-ups. That at least gave me some muscle tone. And the sit-ups were critical at my best running times—when running properly, I feel most effect in my core, running forward instead of the vertical pounding on my back, hips and knees.

Struggling to get back to normal, or my new normal, I am worked on cross-training. At least twice a week, before or after playing tennis, I would spend some time with the girl-sized weights, and my arms felt good. But overall, I was still nowhere near where I thought I should have been.

———

The fitness directive from my EP was to work, slowly, on getting back in shape, but never exceed 150 BPM.

For a couple months I made slow progress. I'd run an HRC (Heart-Rate-Control, not to be confused with a felonious career politician) program on my treadmill. And that was a great measurement tool for me. I set my target at 150, and then spent four or five minutes walking to warm up, and then began running. The treadmill would begin to monitor once I approached within 10% of my target, and the clock would start running toward my goal. Once so triggered, the machine was on cruise control and I was out of the driver's seat. I kept plodding along, and the machine would slow down as necessary to keep me from exceeding my target range.

The difficult variable for me was in the time it would then take me to hit three miles. I was at best, even while working at this for a couple months, only 70% of where I thought I should be (as in where I used to be, pre-op). I did this at home three days a week, and went to the club for the tiny weights and the elliptical, all the while self-monitoring my heart rate and not exceeding my medical prescription.

At about five months post-op, this system broke down. Or maybe my heart became stubborn. Arrhythmia returned, and my treadmill was not happy about it. I could feel it, of course, but tried to power through it (hey, with the monitoring program, I don't over-exert, so I'm cool, right?). But there were several mornings when I would get hooked up, the treadmill would catch my rhythm, and promptly shut down. I'm glad it did not talk—it would have said: "you're at 170, dummy—get off me!" And then my heart rate began regularly spiking during exercise.

Frustration. There's that word again. And it gets more frustrating each year, month, week, day, hour and minute.

Maybe it is in my head by now. Physiological, psychosomatic, whatever—it's here, it's *still* here, and it sucks.

———

When the weather turned spring-like, I was eager to make the treadmill-to-tarmac transition. On this afternoon I took a slightly different route than usual, largely because it kept me in the warm sunlight instead of the cool shadows. As I passed a point where my congenital stubbornness would not allow me a medical time-out or a turnaround to go home, I felt funny. I felt different. I felt really, very not-good.

I looked at my watch. HR 205. Hmm. Even as bad as I felt, I knew that was not right. Let's keep going. I've been cleared to push myself—I can't do any harm. So no problem. Whatever I am feeling will run its course, so to speak.

So I kept going, and I kept feeling worse. 205, 210, 215 the up a hill and I saw 222. I didn't throw in the towel, but I did maintain my slow uphill pace even after the ascent. I plodded along slowly and pulled it into the barn still running upwards of 200.

I was worn out that night. Almost like when Atrial Flutter had clobbered me, *but I could not tell what my heart was doing.* The feeling stuck with me through the week. I was down. I was confused—I had spent years becoming highly-tuned to Fibrillation and Flutter. This was neither. But I felt worse. *A new frustration? Something worse? Something different? I did not know.* I ran my normal schedule, but slowly, and I was admitting to myself that I was becoming worried, curious…that same old song and lousy dance.

I made it through Friday, and was dragging. I was not a fun spouse at the end of the work week. I propped my eyes open through dinner and went to bed very early, hoping that would wash away the newest and multiplying feelings of fatigue.

I awoke early Saturday and had a cup of normal coffee in an effort to give myself some energy to play tennis. But even with a little caffeine, I was a dead-feeling man walking.

I couldn't catch my breath. I could barely see. After each point I was leaning on my racquet, breathing steadily but shallowly, and waiting for my vision to improve. When I would stop after a point, darkness would encroach on the edges of my fields of vision.

And the worst part is that this was not a hard-fought singles match. This was a fun, competitive, but gentlemanly game of doubles. But I was in sorry shape.

I very specifically went through the thought process that I should be playing tennis with a helmet. I had held it together for nearly an hour, keeping my dire situation from my partner and our opponents, but as I worked to catch my breath after each point, my apparently oxygen-deprived brain was trying to preserve itself...by avoiding a concussion. My principal concern was that I was going to pass out and slam my head on the court. And it felt like it could happen at any moment. The black tunnel tightening my vision could slam shut, the wave of clamminess would wash over me and down I'd go. I was trying to pick a good point in the match when I could run (yeah, right, run) up to the front desk and ask to borrow a bicycle helmet. *It made sense, again, inside of my head—but would they have let me play, after I described my situation? How I needed a helmet because I thought I was going to pass out because I've got a heart "problem?" Not smart.*

I did finally smarten up, and at the end of the second set, I quit. "Guys—I'm sorry to let you down, but I cannot go on. My heart is feeling funny—no nothing to worry about, but I feel very bad. This time, I'm afraid, discretion is going to be the better part of valor."

They were of course understanding and concerned about me. I took a cup of coffee on the way out, eager that the caffeine would drive me for my ten-minute trip home. One friend was concerned about me driving, but he strangely believed my incoherent protestations: "I'm not worried about it when I am consistently seated, like when driving. The worrisome part is when I start and stop, like playing tennis, or when I sit and rise (like I will need to do to get out of the car at home, but I can catch the garage wall if necessary)."

"Okay, Adam—drive safely, and I hope you feel better. We'll look forward to seeing you next week."

I made it home fine. I did grab the garage wall and the car door when I had to dismount. I said hello, immediately parked myself on the couch…and stayed there nearly all weekend. I was in sorry shape. I could not keep my eyes open. I did not walk the dog, I did not read. I only dozed through hazy television shows, ate dinner, slept overnight, and repeated (without the leaving the house for physical activity nonsense) on Sunday.

Another Failure, A Bigger Sledgehammer

MONDAY MORNING I was on the hotline again. I spoke to several nice nurses as they chased my doctor around the building. A few return calls later, and they asked me to take it easy, but self-monitor for several days. If I still felt lousy, they'd bring me in for an ECG, and maybe hook me in to a Holter monitor. And that's what we did for that week.

My kindly local guys fit me in. The tests were conclusive. "Yes, no wonder you feel poorly. You are now in what is called Junctional Rhythm."

"Hmm, I haven't heard of that one…but I gather it's not good."

"Well, you have your (next) ablation planned at the end of next month, don't you? I would strongly urge you to not exert yourself until then."

"That's about six weeks. I've been patient, and yet eager to get back to a normal life. The sun is shining, and I want to move my bones. But you're saying nothing? For more than a month and a half?" "Why am I still going through this?!?!?!"

Frustration. A new frustration.

———

Study Result
Narrative

Pat Name: ADAM EHLERT Department: CARD
Patient ID: Room:
Gender: Male Technician: A45677
DOB: 1973-02-15 Requested By: Dr. M
Order Number: 174255268
Measurements
Intervals Axis
Rate: 38 P:
PR: QRS: 6
QRSD: 86 T: 53
QT: 516
QTc: 411
Interpretive Statements
SINUS BRADYCARDIA
Compared to ECG 02/18/2016 07:49:34
Junctional rhythm now present
Sinus bradycardia no longer present
Ventricular premature complex(es) no longer present
T-wave abnormality no longer present

———

Junctional Rhythm feels like Bradycardia on Quaaludes.

I felt awful. I could not function, and it quickly became apparent that my blood was not flowing, northward nor southward. My brain and energy felt compromised. And physically, my legs and ankles were swelling. I couldn't believe it! When I wore socks, it would take all evening for any elastic seam marks to be flushed from my skin. And if I was seated with my calf against a table leg, the imprint would stay there for hours.

This was actually worse. Worse, worse, worse than any Atrial Fibrillation. I was always down, drained, exhausted. The moment I woke up was the best I felt all day. One step downstairs began the worry and growing fatigue.

To this day I still practice, unintentionally, small acts of self-preservation that have been conditioned over my years of lightheadedness. The simplest is that I tap one heel on the top of the top step before I start a descent. If one is already unease afoot, a misstep at the top can cause a fright…or a fall. And that's a tough way to get your blood moving. I don't recall a conscious step (so to speak) to start this tic, but I know it is a simple confirmation of where the steps begin, and where I am in relation.

———

Junctional Rhythm is a sort of failsafe for the body. Thank goodness for that. A normal beat is triggered by a sequential electrical signal—the current begins at the SA Node, in the upper part of the heart. This contracts the atria. The signal then travels downward to the AV Node, which causes the ventricles to contract. Sequential: buh-bump, buh-bump, over and over and over. Poe's madman described it as a "low, dull, quick sound," a description with which I cannot argue. And yet I might be qualified to be such a judge, as my own was driving me crazy.

The sequence of the electrical signals is what allows the upper and lower chambers to fill and empty in full, and in proper order. In Junctional Rhythm, the "beat" signals come from the AV node, exclusively. There are several potential reasons for this. One is called "Sick Sinus Syndrome." I believe that's when your Sino-Arial Node conks out. It can also be "caused," either via a surgical slip (which I highly doubt in my case, and especially several months later as they've cured it after multiple examinations), or pharmacologically. A combination of drugs—both rate control and/or rhythm control—can have perhaps more than the desired (and less targeted) effect. This can inhibit the SA Node from firing. Or, occasionally and for no reason at all, that chief semaphore can just "get sleepy."

No matter the cause, it is reassuring to have a redundant system. This system, however, does not work as efficiently as the original design. When all signals *start* at the AV node, there is no *sequence.* In a simple description, the electrical trigger signal radiates outward to all four chambers simultaneously. They all contract, or beat, but not effectively nor sequentially. The fill-empty-fill-empty sequence does not happen. The blood continues to flow in the proper direction, but with only little whispers of flow with each "beat."

The lack of real flow is why I had no energy, was always sleepy, was unable to recover from even moderate activity (like having my legs underneath my chair).

I did follow doctors' orders, and did nothing for about six weeks. It was a drag, but as I was dragging myself, I was frankly glad to have the shut-down order from on high. Otherwise I would have felt guilty and tried to keep pushing myself. I would have remained steadfast in my reckless belief that energy begets energy

———

As with persistent Atrial Fibrillation, the fatigue is cumulative—at least for me, anyway. With Junctional Rhythm, I started the day feeling poorly, and got worse as the day dragged on. I started Monday as rested as possible, and grew worse as each day in the week wore on.

Thank goodness I had a late-June relief plan.

———

Once more we loaded up and traversed the beautiful (really) state of Iowa, which must have the safest freeways in the union. I think the unofficial state motto is: "Iowa—the state where achieving the speed limit is an impossible dream!"

Here we are again, with the Monday-Tuesday, prep-and-go plan. This was to be my (next) latest and greatest salvation. A simple ablation. Simple for me, anyway. As Dr. S had described months ago, the chances for success were decent, as were the chances that he could simply access the needed areas. Because I already had scar tissue in the heart, outside of the heart…oh, and the little closure device smack dab in the middle of the heart, this "simple" procedure might be a little more complicated.

He could do it. And by that I mean that HE could do it. Not that I was averse to a road game, and I still had utmost confidence in the Pros from Dover, but a local option was not even an option. The trick is that one has to go up and around the closure device. It *can be* done, but no local physician had ever done it. Dr. S has done several dozen. At the March meeting, he described the intricate procedure, he offered that it might take eight to 10 hours. To which I flippantly responded: "What do I care? You're the one doing all the work." He smoothly glossed past my opprobriousness. Later in the day I realized that duration might affect my recovery. But I still looked forward to it.

As Monday arrived, we ran through the usual protocol. I had a number of tests, starting in the early morning. Heather caught up to me in the early afternoon, before they juiced me for a TEE. I'm sure I was to be glad to have an escort as I awoke. All was on schedule, and I stumbled out about 3:30. My morning report time was again at for "Group A," so we planned an early dinner. Heather had even made reservations for a 5:30 table on the patio at the place next door to our hotel. Great—early dinner, back for the soap-up, into bed early and back at it before the crack of dawn.

Back in the hotel I sent some "final" messages, tried to watch a baseball game, but later realized it was a replay of the previous night's (I should have known the Twins could not win two in a row that summer), and put on a sweater for our dinner al fresco.

As I had one arm into the sweater (it might have taken me a while, as I was still loopy from the brief anesthetization), my phone rang.

CALL ID: Mayo Clinic, Rochester, MN.
"Adam, this is Dr. S. I am working on my preparations for tomorrow, and am going over today's imaging. Have you ever had any kidney problems?"

"Um...huh? No." "What do you mean?"

"Well, I see a spot at the top of one; it's your right kidney. I really cannot tell exactly what it is, and so I was hoping you could tell me if you had had any history. Absent that, I have already sent it to Dr. N, and to the head of our Urology Department, and to the head Radiologist. We will work tonight to determine its origin and nature. We'll see you tomorrow."

"Um, okay. Do I need to worry about this? Do I still report as if we are proceeding at as scheduled (precisely twelve hours from now)?"

"I am not able to answer for sure any specifics about the image I am seeing. But we will have clarity before we do anything. Yes, go ahead and come in tomorrow morning, as planned."

"Um, okay. Thank you for calling, doctor."

———

"Heather—that was Dr. S. He asked if I had ever had any kidney problems. He sees something in today's imaging. But he told me to not worry, and he will see us in the morning."

"What?!"

"He told me to not worry, but he did not say it very vigorously. I'm maybe a little worried...but there's nothing I can do."

"Let's hurry up and eat and hurry up and sleep, and we'll work toward resolution in the morning."

Worry. Fatigue. Frustration.

———

PAGING PATIENT TWO

It was a beautiful summer afternoon, and I was looking forward to the early dinner, outside, and just across the street. I was still reeling from the drugs two hours ago, and more reeling from the phone call four minutes ago. As we stepped across the sidewalk, I suggested that I would wait outside. Our table was to be out here, and the fully able-bodied one could navigate the stream of happy-hour-goers, check in at the host stand, and I'd hold up the light post outside and out of the way.

Good plan, lousy execution. Heather was quickly back by my side, but something had changed. And it was not good.

She had opened the exterior door right onto/into her big toe's toenail. She ripped that sucker almost all the way off. And whether it was fully off, or just dangling, it was spurting bright red blood.

At least I forgot about my heart. And my kidney.

I did have the wherewithal to stumble in and appeal for a stack of paper napkins. We then, Tweedle-Drugged and Tweedle-Clumsy hobbled across the main street, right up the steps to Saint Mary's Hospital. A massive building, from which doctors, interns, nurses and students were streaming, as it was about 5:32.

Being a hospital, I knew it would house wheelchairs, whether or not we found immediate help. We did not, but I dumped my lovely and crippled wife in a chair, and wheeled her in a near-straight line down each hallway, simply following all of the bright red "EMERGENCY" way finders.

What a pair! What a sight. My normally-graceful but now-angst-ridden wife rolling down the hospital hallways holding a bloody wad of cocktail napkins on her big toe, and me, half-stoned, listing and wobbling down those hallways, following the big red signs.

It is a good thing that our opinion of the Mayo Clinic was already well established before we served time in the Emergency Room. It is not their strong suit.

Part of it may have been because of our messaging. We were in an honest-to-God-place-for-real-emergencies. And at face value, we were not one. By all rights, we should have been at a Minute Clinic or Urgent Care. Barring that, there is another hospital, with frankly a much better ER on the outskirts of town. But it was really difficult for the clerks to understand that we could not get there.

As I wheeled her forward to the glass-enclosed triage station, Heather naturally spoke up first. She was nine toes ahead of me, and I was halfway in outer space anyway. Somehow, all they heard was "stubbed toenail." Their closed ears only furthered Heather's frustration, and I certainly was not going to be able to communicate any more effectively. I was there to not crash the wheelchair into things, and to procure paper napkins as necessary.

After a while and after a mini-rush (of a child's summertime broken arm, a drunk driving accident instigator, a softball accident victim, surrounded by sock-and-slide-wearing 12-year old girls, and a delegation from the eastern-bloc Tuberculosis transmission committee), the clerks seemed to notice the incongruity of this healthy but confusing couple of 40-year-olds. Especially the "non-ER-patient" husband, who strangely was already wearing his own complement of Mayo wristbands.

After four hours she was seen. Yes, four (Heather—they really do need to care for that gunshot wound victim, even though you were here first) hours. I do not fault the delay, but the tough part was that the waiting room was not clean. It was uncomfortably filthy and gross.

During those long 240 minutes, Heather vacillated of course between feeling angry at the slow wheels of emergency room care, and worriedly advocating for me, the lightly-incapacitated, short-on-sleep patient-to-be. Yeah—the guy who hasn't eaten all day. She only infrequently felt sorry for herself. Halfway in (but we didn't know if halfway) she did phone the restaurant to ask for a to-go club sandwich...and to cancel our blood-stained reservation. I dutifully crisscrossed the corridors and then scampered across the street ("rush" hour having long past), to retrieve my meal and then eat it while perched on the cleanest corner of ER couch I could find. Good—some nourishment before the long day tomorrow. Thank you, my dear.

Once she was ushered back, the medical professionals were of course wonderful. They understood how it happened (and yes, they chuckled, sympathetic to our situation) they understood Heather's cosmetic concern for the nail (this is a woman who wears sandals whenever possible and above 20 degrees), and they did everything they could to ensure its salvation. They were great and we hobbled/wobbled out of there around 11:00 pm.

Across the street, clean up, and sleep fast! On the bright side, no real time to stew with worry about my kidney "situation."

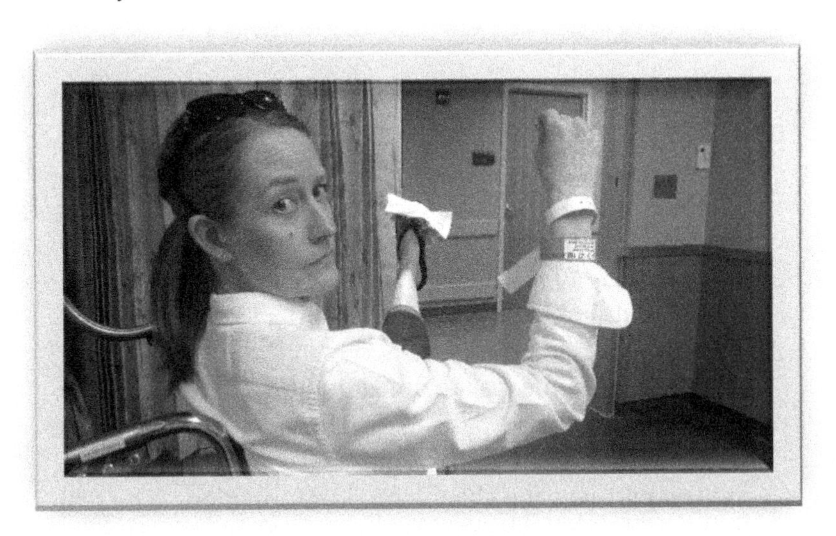

The Next Last Procedure?

5:25 AM: WE WALK across the street and in the hospital's main entrance. It was dark, so I could not check the grand front steps for 11-hour-old bloodstains. I'm lined up inside for admission and all goes smoothly.

They usher me back, update some vitals, perforate both forearms…and park me in a closet. To wait, and wait, and wait. I think Tom Petty was wrong—the hardest part was the sheer lack of information. The real irony is that simple communication—almost as important as the specific doctoring itself—is a hallmark of the Mayo patient's experience. Don't get me wrong. In my heart of hearts, I know I was not being neglected—there were cardiologists and urologists and radiologists swirling all around. But not one of them circled back to me with so much as "we're on it." This was at least four hours. I may have victimized myself by a conscious decision to not bring the book I was reading. I was traveling light—I didn't need a book taking up valuable space in my medical commuter's belongings bag. And so I sat there idly. Idly stewing. Idly worrying.

Or almost idly. My closet did have a television…circa 1986. Likely it was my frustrated and distracted state of mind, but the television was almost more frustration than it was worth. It was mounted at funny angle in the corner of the room, hanging from the ceiling. I had an ancient four-button remote control on the end of a garden hose, and the screen was about ten inches diagonal. On the bright side, it received more than six channels, but I never really made it far through the list because it took about seven seconds for a one-step change to happen. I looked at this TV, in this tiny room, a lot…but I did not enjoy any of it. But I know it was my state of mind. In that condition, I would not have enjoyed the sweeping drama and landscapes of *Lonesome Dove* even on a 65-inch monstrosity. I could have, however, cycled through all six hours…many times over.

———

After four-plus hours, a haggard-looking Dr. S strode down the hall. I was wandering looking for a bathroom mostly out of boredom, but was happy to return to the outhouse-sized staging room for his report. He did report, but he did not know anything. They had no real definition on the kidney curiosity. And as scientists, they did not feel good about proceeding without proper data and knowledge of all variables.

I was glad to hear that. What did it mean to me? Long term…and especially short-term? Much like the arrhythmia marathon itself, my recent 24 hours had spun me to be tired, hungry, curious, frustrated…and a new, weightier emotion—I was frightened.

The day became a blur, mostly of inactivity and mounting vexation. They kept me cooped up in the coop for a few more hours. Mostly, I understand, because they did not have a proper place for me. I was not in the operating theater, as had been scheduled for 8-10 hours. Nor could they put me in a real recovery room, meant for real, recovering patients.

I was finally moved (t*hey* moved *me*—I was not allowed to walk) to what I hoped was a new but temporary home. It was a multi-person room. And I know I will sound like an entitled prima donna here, but it was a harsh awakening, but made me think compassionately. Compassionately later, anyway, once we got through this dragging exasperation.

My in-patient experiences had been fairly sterile to-date. Traumatic at times, but most often very clean, boring and the only stress being generated principally inside my own head. As a rule, "cardiac patients" are generally placed in private rooms, unless requested otherwise by the patient or the patient's insurer. Trying to balance my own foibles with those of some other person, some other *sick person*, were outside the bounds of what I could reconcile, or even simply handle at the moment. Combined with the aforementioned fatigue, hunger, curiosity, newfound fear and ubiquitous frustration, and I was on an emotional disaster course.

We'd been through the bulk of the afternoon. I think. It's funny, in recollection, this date feels like a mid-winter one. Probably because I was up and in before the dawn, having never seen the light of day. This was June, in the upper Midwest, where it stays light late. But when I was parked in the inboard bed (close to the room's door, away from the window; good for airplanes, bad for hospitals), I had a vague cognizance of dusk out the distant embrasure.

So I figured I had been incarcerated for 16 hours at least. I had next-to-no information. And I wanted a little bit of ice water. And when a nurse who was maybe not ready for me forgot my simple request, three times, I ashamedly got ugly. Stress can lower one's personal expectations for behavior.

I'm not ashamed that I acted, or over-reacted. I am glad because it did spur some action. I'm almost disappointed in myself that I attacked the nurse directly…but only almost. I know I asked very politely the first two times, and then offered a friendly reminder the third time. It is a small matter, but when one simple component of a patient's comfort—never mind one simple request directly from the patient's mouth itself—is ignored or forgotten, something is wrong. I suspect the poor girl was simply not paying attention. The silver lining though, is that I got to apologize later on, allow her to understand what brought on my anger, and from then on she paid attention to every syllable. She even bonded with Heather, commiserating for me, and trying to accommodate other requests as a priority. That spousal commiseration led my new advocate to understand what a long day it had been, and that a shared room would not be pleasant for anyone. Heather did not say this threateningly, but maybe as a caution to the staff that the wearied patient she knows so well was not comfortable (and then makes everyone else less-so).

Two things happened pretty quickly. A convention was called surrounding my bed (and there was plenty of room as my mate had not yet arrived), chaired by a very senior-ranking physician, and the staff on my floor decided to ask forgiveness instead of permission, and moved me to the held-out-for-a-potential-VIP room down the hall. It was not a special room, but I think they do need to keep some in reserve for special or concerning cases. I had no compunction about being that particular patient at that particular time.

The convened medical team was there to answer any questions, and take any slings and arrows if necessary. I was cordial (mostly, perhaps), but recounted my concerns frustrations and agony. Nobody offered any platitudes, and nor should they have. But the team leader described the medical limbo I was in, the steps they were looking at toward direction, and the parts that the various departments and professionals were taking toward that direction.

This very quickly became very serious. From their intensity I took gravity and fear.

It was a useful meeting. The air was cleared. We were collectively on the same page.

The "plan" was to seek greater definition on my kidney. We'd handle that variable, and then shift back to my heart. I was to try to get some sleep. My first nurse was falling all over herself to ensure great care, and I was doing the same to show appreciation. The handoff to the night crew was done with some substance, too. My superstar night nurse pre-coordinated the timing of my last medications and monitoring, and then placed a very cordial "Do Not Disturb" sign on my door. I got nearly six hours of sleep, and then imaging and tests began anew in the morning.

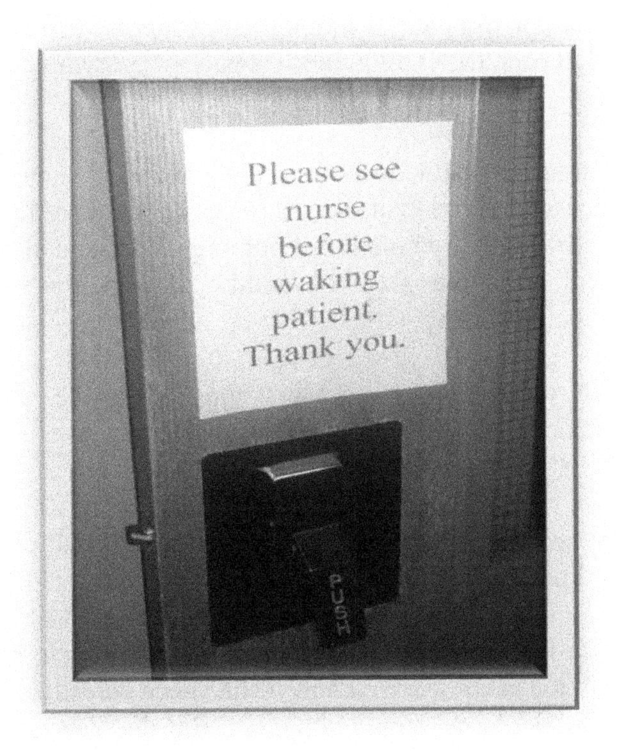

Long story short, it took a day and a half to get to a "we don't really know anything specifically, be we feel secure that your kidney should not impede any heart procedure" statement. This was *after* a tough meeting with a very straightforward urologist. The gist of which was that my kidney's curious growth looked like a tumor, in all likelihood malignant. They would watch it closely, gain another set of data points in two months when they looked again (at Mayo, so I could be seen on the exact same machines, calibrated the exact same way), and determine the action plan then. Likely a biopsy, and likely removal of the darn thing—either immediately that day or after three months, six months, or even a couple years, depending upon its pace of growth.

———

A long, stressful, do-nothing day. We had planned on a successful ablation at the very-capable hands of Dr. S. Instead we got a whole lot of nothing. Worse, actually, we got a whole slew of additional concerns—one principally starting with "C."

We were reeling. We were trying to breathe. I had had exactly one soggy turkey sandwich for sustenance over 36 hours.

We were reminding each other to be thankful of the serendipitous timing of this discovery.

And Dr. N walked in the room. It must have been 8:00 in the evening. We knew he had been consulted and kept "in the loop" on my situation. But this was not his situation. It was not his area of expertise. It was not his responsibility.

He could not add anything.

But he did. He made everything better, that very instant. He smiled. My wife burst into tears the like I have never seen from her. He shook my hand. He hugged Heather.

He was our Alpha and Omega. This was pure human altruism. *Care.* All would be alright.

At the end of his long day, he took the few extra steps to track down my room and simply say hello.

Everyday care for him. Life-altering emotion and reassurance for this couple from Kansas.

———

C is for Cookies

Rochester, MN 9:00 PM
(Email to my family, from a hospital bed after two very long days—aborted ablation, Pacemaker planned, likely Cancer diagnosis (but I couldn't at the time bring myself to write that word).

I love cookies. And I could maybe finagle one for myself now, but I'm torn. I've got three hours before "NOTHING to eat or drink," but I really don't want to gorge myself right up to the deadline. I'll relish more the recovery treat afterwards if I eat reasonably beforehand.

It's been a rough couple days/weeks/months and years. I've burned through a lot of frustration, and I've also gained a great deal of perspective. Especially lately.

———

Right now I'm sitting in a hospital room, wholly inactive, in more ways than one. I've been sitting, and waiting, and doing nothing for two days straight. I've got IVs in both arms. When the phlebotomist asked a nurse to turn off my left IV so that she could perforate that arm further and take blood, the nurse promptly turned off the right one. In her defense, it was her left, but I thought the patient always came first, perhaps, though, except in areas of directional nursing.

———

But moving on from my service malaise, this was a day of activity. Not all great, but the fact that there was activity and communication made it a marked improvement over the prior day.

Today's nice contrast to yesterday, and also my coming few days was that I spent most of it out of bed—purely for variety. The bed is differently-uncomfortable than the hospital room chairs. And at least the bed moves.

Yesterday started with great enthusiasm (as much enthusiasm as one with a half-functioning heart can muster in the pre-dawn half-light). We recognized the wake-up call, cleaned up, put on dirty clothes, and jaywalked across the street into Saint Mary's Hospital. I really enjoyed the clockwork fashion of the opening ceremonies—first report time is 5:30, and as we lined up like we were boarding a Southwest Airlines flight, the clerks filed out at exactly 5:27:30, and flipped their signs and called up the front of the lines right at 5:30 on the button.

About five minutes after registration, I was led upstairs to a prep room. They did some last-minute paperwork, stabbed me in both forearms, and then said they'd get back to me. And then nothing. For four hours. It was agonizing.

Plans change.

———

You see, Dr. S called me on Monday night. He asked, at about 4:30, if I had ever experienced any kidney problems? He was reviewing all imaging in advance of the Tuesday morning procedure, and saw something that puzzled him. My right kidney did not look right. He told me he had called Dr. N already, and also had a call in to my Internist at Executive Health, Dr. D. Nope—no history, whistle-clean blood tests from a scant three months ago, and never any concern.

Dr. S is a cardiologist. A spectacular cardiologist. Perhaps, like anything, it is preparation and attention to detail that makes one great. That, with the conviction in one's own knowledge, coupled with an unwavering desire to do right for the patient makes one a truly spectacular physician. Dr. S began pursuing answers and expert opinions. From colleagues as zealous and devoted as he is to his specialty.

His devotion made for a tough Tuesday for yours truly. I had been worried about the wearying effect of an 8-10-hour procedure. Granted, I did not have to do anything beyond lying stock-still, in an undoubtedly chilly operating theater, and under serious anesthesia for that long would be, in a word, exhausting.

But the waiting and wondering and growing frustrated was worse. A lot worse. Mostly because of the uncertainty. By late Tuesday, we agreed: the ablation was off, we'd eventually default to a much safer (in more ways than one) Pacemaker installation, and we would wait to hear from and discuss with, Urology and Radiology—there was a chance they might want to do an MRI, and that is better done before implanting a small computer with wires attaching to my heart.

Dr. S' primary concern was the unknown properties of the kidney "image." The ablation is an involved and technical procedure, and, owing to my previous heart vagaries, involves thinning my blood down to about the viscosity of college beer. If the kidney "thing" was going to bleed, there was next to nothing he could do about it—especially with a needle lodged in my atrial septum.

Tuesday through Tuesday night was a very scary time.

So we delayed. And on Wednesday morning got a nice report (through the cardiac rhythm team) from the Urology specialists. In its current form, which I guess is all we have, the kidney mass cannot hurt me. It is only about half the size of any cyst or tumor that would grow or metastasize aggressively. And we need a second data point to understand how quickly it is growing, if at all—there was a chance that it's been with me for years, and could also be a byproduct of my congenital heart problems.

And so we move forward. There is no need for an MRI, therefore the Pacemaker can be done at any time. And the option was "maybe sometime" on Wednesday—they could put me on the list, or, second-thing on Thursday morning. Thursday morning was a better option—everyone is fresh, Dr. S can do it himself, and I can breathe and eat and relax (yeah, right), through Wednesday.

———

I did get to eat. Three meals, and I'm learning what hospitals can do well, and what their limitations may be. Breakfast can be pretty good. Lunch also. Soups are somewhat safe, and the trick is to stay away from the dinner-entrée items. Lukewarm and bland and gelatinous are not desirable characteristics for chicken or fish. Dinner was again an egg-salad sandwich, a cup of soup, some cottage cheese and a small but excellent chocolate milkshake—my third in four meals (I withheld for breakfast).

So Wednesday was meals and meetings and a learning curve. The first report from the cardiac rhythm team did give me a little peace of mind, and also allowed for a plan to move forward. Clear direction—pacemaker in the morning.

The plan was good, and the learning was necessary, unfortunately. Or perhaps better—fortunately and with deep, grounded appreciation.

———

The Urologist came to discuss in the afternoon. He walked us through what he knew, what he had discussed with and learned from his colleagues, and what it meant to me. He was clear, concise, and candid. He shared a great deal of information, all the while walking a tight line between overwhelming technical stuff, and translating it to be useful to my spinning head.

It turns out that, even as the jingle goes, "C" is not only for cookies. We'd had, until now, a lot of conjecture and speculation about cysts and tumors, malignant and benign. But at the early stages, and without any starkly definitive smoking gun, it didn't mean much.

Even now, I've heard the word, but I'm not sure it's sunk in. I really can't yet bring myself to say it. I guess I can describe the diagnosis, and maybe I can do that because it is still so early, and not fully defined.

The "cyst" does not look like a cyst (which would be inherently benign). Yes, it's way too early to make any predictions, dire or otherwise, but it does not look like a cyst. Therefore, dear Watson, it looks like a tumor.

What we'll do is watch it. I'll be under active observation. And it'll happen here, at Mayo. I'm scheduled for another (another, another) CT scan in a couple months. One early conversation indicated that I could do the scan anywhere, and the information would be sent no problem to my Mayo team. The Urologist indicated otherwise, in no uncertain terms. I'll visit Rochester again, have the imaging done on the same machines, calibrated in the same way, and will have full consultation with the Urology, Radiology, and Cookie(?) teams. And heck—I can have a little follow up on my bionic-to-be heart at the same time!

The second set of images will give us, most importantly, a second data point. Is it growing, and how fast? Cysts and tumors grow differently and at different paces...and this is clearly not a cyst.

I don't yet have the Urologist's candor. Nor can I use the specific word he used. But I sure am thinking about it.

———

I am thankful for a lot of things.

The doctors of course are spectacular. Even that old sawbones Dr. H—if my "mother of all open-heart surgeries" had worked a year ago, I would not be back here. Today. And Dr. S would have not performed his diligence in looking at each and every speck on every bit of film. And maybe technology is part of the solution? If the imaging was constricted by literal film, it may not have run an inch or so low, capturing the top of my kidneys. But how was it not seen three months ago, when they had to take extra images, burning extra X-Ray film, to capture all of my "long" lungs?

I'm not going to run through all the what-ifs. There are too many, on both sides of the ledger. But really only the one that matters. I'm amazed and thankful that Dr. S looked outside of his scope. I'm thankful I'm here.

I'm thankful for Heather, and especially her perspective and support throughout. Her spontaneous, sincere and enthusiastic waterworks when Dr. N walked through my door last night remains one of my best memories of this particular medical tour. And much, much, much more so I am thankful for her perspective on my renal discovery. It is serendipitous and remarkable that the stars have aligned for this little and life-altering fork in the road.

———

I'm not really happy about "it," whatever it may be. But until three months from now, when we have a better idea, I am going to cling to the idea that "C is for Cookies." And that sureashell is good enough for me.

To Be Bionic

SO, WE'RE BACK to concentrating on the known organ, my heart. Dr. S was cleared to work his magic, in whatever direction he chose. And we were back at a decision point. The plan had been for an ablation. A very intricate one that would take a long time. The determinant in this direction was that it was another step toward amelioration, before more drastic steps would be needed. In short, the ablation could fix my symptoms. The more drastic step, a Pacemaker, would also likely fix my symptoms…but I'd also be beholden to the thing for the rest of my life.

But as my delay had worn on (mind you, I was in misery-inducing Junctional Rhythm throughout), Dr S changed course. He was worried about my simple walking-around ability, and amazed, frankly, that I was not passing out on a regular basis from the junctional effects or simple bradycardia. And so, my fix shifted from the planned ablation, to the installation of a Pacemaker.

The Pacer was to be a good move for a couple of reasons: 1) it was to keep me beating at the level of a normal, living person, and 2) it has a rhythm-control feature (!!!). *It is of note that, I would soon learn that the "rhythm control" therapy is not bulletproof (compared to my stubborn heart, anyway).* Most significant is that they installed an *MRI-compatible* device, owing to my impending kidney transactions.

———

The procedure was pretty simple. And I remember waking with a monitor directly over my bed. It was flashing: "65…65…65…six-ty-five…six-ty-five…six-ty-five…." I had not seen that consistent of a number in what felt like years. It was hypnotic. I was enthralled. Calm, but enthralled nonetheless.

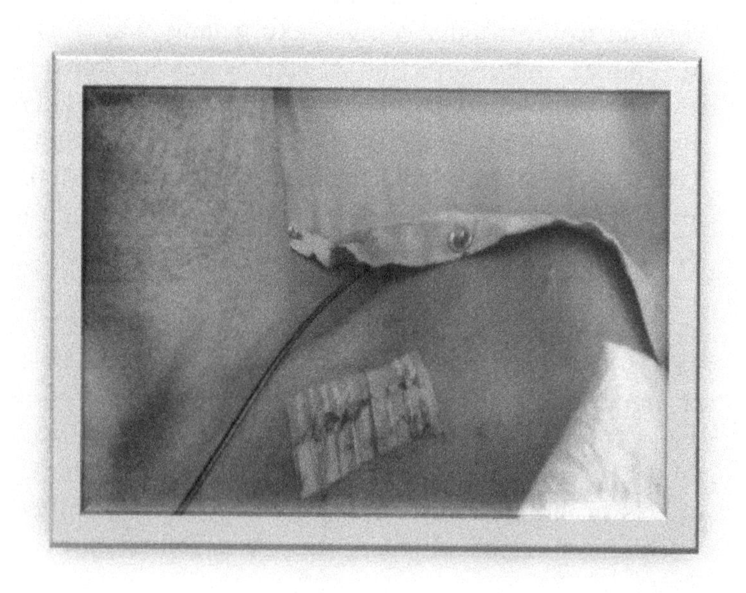

I stayed in the hospital that night, and woke up pushing for information and progress. Things moved remarkably quickly.

Dr. S came by for a final check. His team worked on coordinating my local follow-up and my follow-up back in Rochester in two months. The Urology team did the same.

As our final consultation was at midday, I was offered the opportunity to leave that afternoon. It was give and take, and solely dependent upon how I felt. "I feel like I'm already halfway down I-35!" "Alright, we'll begin discharge paperwork." "Wait—you're not driving, right?"

Medtronic is watching, Danica

Speaking of driving...we made it home for the holiday weekend, which was nice because it allowed me to actually catch my breath and not try to recuperate too quickly. The Pacemaker procedure really was fairly simple (three-inch bloody gash notwithstanding), but I think the heaviness of my three-day stay was the most fatiguing overall. Stress is wearying.

Heather succumbed to the Red Mist on the trip home. As the GPS calculator presents a "time at destination," a competitive person naturally begins to try to beat it. We made it, and were home before 8:30.

Two days later I conducted my Pacemaker's first "handshake." This is when I send a transmission via my bedside machine, and it communicates with the computers at the mother ship. The transmission looked like it was going out properly from my machine. A few minutes later I called to check if received: "Yes, Mr. Ehlert, I see it coming through just fine."

Two hours later: "Hello Mr. Ehlert—this is Mayo Rhythm Services. We spoke a couple hours ago. As I look closely at your transmission, I see a couple of episodes of elevated heart rate, upwards of 150, at two times two days ago. Can I ask—do you recall what you were doing at 2:30 and again at about 5:15?"

"Um, yes, at 2:30 I was just checking out of the hospital—I guess I was eager to leave." And at 5:15 I was a couple hours down the interstate. I guess my wife was eager to get home. I promise you that she is really

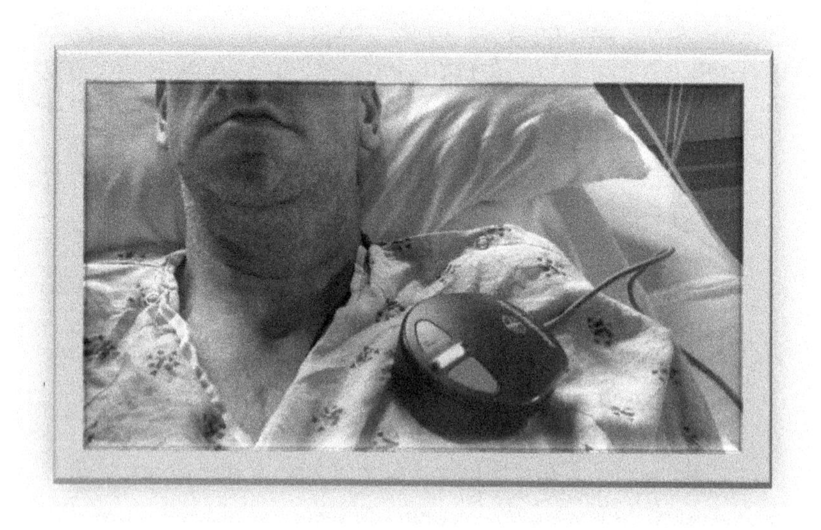

a good driver, but I am glad you are monitoring me—I will ask her to slow down in the future, thank you."

———

July 2, (email to my brothers)

Zach and Nate--a little more information:

I am home, sort of resting. Heather tried to set a new Minnesota-to-Kansas land speed record yesterday, and I am glad for it.

I was a little slow sharing information this week. Largely because it was changing quickly, and partially because it was tough to sink in my thick skull (combined with a stubborn Ehlert heart).

Long story short: the path we had chosen for this current heart procedure was fraught with variables. We had a pretty good understanding of them after consultation with Dr. S on Monday afternoon. The variables multiplied however, when he spotted—purely by happenstance—something on my kidney. This discovery changed cardiac variables to, literally and figuratively, the path of least resistance, hence Pacemaker.

More heart work will need to be done, but not right now. The Pacemaker gets me out of immediate danger. And then the priority goes back to the" incidental-oma" on my kidney.

I'm not at any impending risk, and we'll get a better handle on it in a couple months. It was pure luck they spotted it, and there was nothing I should have done additionally or differently. Nor, frankly, should you.

Call if you'd like to discuss, anytime. I'm sorry I have not yet, but it's still sinking in.

Thanks, love,
Adam

———

I was home. I had my new technological salvation healing in my upper chest. I was optimistic…and I perhaps naively assumed that I would get used to the Pacer's bulk (still not yet). The small protrusion below my collarbone would cure my Bradycardia, Junctional Rhythm and perpetual fear of falling down dark.

But things take time. I had a "wound check" with my GP at home. I then days later had a Pacer check in my Cardiology Practice office. *"So, I was told that it might take a few days to dial in the Atrial Rhythm Therapy feature. Can you do that?"* …Blank look from the check-in aide… *"You see, I am still having a significant number of accelerated rate episodes. My Owner's Manual states that it is best to wait about 10 days for the Pacer itself and especially the leads, to root and become secure, before turning on the reverse-zap feature. Can you do it now?"*

So yes, I was overly-optimistic, or just continually naïve. It takes time. And as I consider retrospectively, my heart takes time to 'calm down' from any procedure. My disappointment from the tuning technician waned with time. I exercised every day, but not as aggressively as I'd have liked. Partially because I was due back to Mayo in just two months. I would then get direction on my kidney cancer, and would also get my Pacer re-tuned. And partially because I had "why bother?" perpetually running through the back of my mind.

———

August: back to Rochester. We had the usual battery of tests and post-test consultations.

I learned that "tuning" my Pacemaker is not an automatic. And...more *frustratingly*, that the Rhythm Control feature is not always effective in every patient. Guess who might be the difficult one?

I now consider that my heart is especially sensitive to being poked and prodded. It probably took these two months for it to stabilize. So now, months later when this team of technicians dialed me in, it was much more effective. I could actively feel as they spun it up toward 100 bpm, and then of course as it was brought back to my hopeful-normal 65...65...65...six-ty-five.

I *almost* take back some of my local frustration at their inability to make it work after a mere 10 days.

My heart was (now) great. On to other organs. We saw two doctors sequentially. The first was a studious, explain-every-detail resident. But he was wonderfully direct and efficient when it came time to deliver the news: "there was no reason to worry." I know he said a bunch more technical stuff after that, but my mind was blank, and I was simply enjoying the tears streaming from Heather's bright blue eyes.

8/30 NOTE

HISTORY OF PRESENT ILLNESS ***Mr. Ehlert is a very pleasant, 43-year-old gentleman*** *whom I saw at the request of Dr. R. for the above complaint.* ***Mr. Ehlert has treatment-refractory atrial fibrillation and atrial flutter. He has undergone multiple procedures for the same.*** *He had a CTA of the chest in June which showed an exophytic right renal mass. The ultrasound was done in follow up and remained indeterminate. A CT of the abdomen and pelvis from June was concerning for cystic renal neoplasm. He is seen today with follow up CT abdomen for discussion of renal mass. He is asymptomatic from this including flank pain or gross hematuria. He does have some symptoms from his cardiac difficulties including shortness of breath and fatigue.* ***His ablation from June was postponed, and they elected for pacemaker placement due to this renal mass.***

IMAGING I personally reviewed the CT imaging as well as the ultrasound focusing on this renal mass. On CT abdomen from August 30, noncontrast view, shows thickened cystic wall without enhancement, and no appreciable change since previous CT scan.

IMPRESSION #1 Bosniak IIF cyst #2 Treatment-refractory arrhythmia #3 Chronic anticoagulation with

Eliquis #4 Status post dual-chamber pacemaker placement June 30, #5 Status post open MAZE procedure for treatment of A fib July 28, #6 Status post ASD closure.

I had the pleasure of meeting with Mr. Ehlert and his wife in the office today along with Dr. T. today. We discussed his renal lesion. We discussed cystic renal lesions as well as small renal masses. We discussed that given this is a cyst which is stable at two-month imaging, we could follow it in 6 to 12 months. This could be done with ultrasound versus CT. They would like to repeat a renal ultrasound in six months which would be March or April and then plan to come back for Executive Health. We discussed bleeding risks for this, and he would be at no higher risk than somebody without a renal cyst. The renal cyst would not preclude any other procedures or anticoagulation. All of their questions were answered. Thank you very much for this consultation.

PATIENT EDUCATION Ready to learn, no apparent learning barriers were identified; learning preferences include listening. Explained diagnosis and treatment plan; patient expressed understanding of the content.

The Patient's Perspective

WHEN MY SAGA began, I had the benefit (?) of having never had any major physical problems, nor any surgeries, elective or otherwise.

I question the benefit because I had no base of knowledge with which to work or prepare or compare. As I consider now, several years in, I do think that was a positive…only because I was pleasantly naive going in. Part of my logic in chronicling my story is to help the more than 25% of Americans who will be affected by Atrial Fibrillation have some sort of an idea what to expect.

Mind you—my case is abnormal for a few different reasons.

We think my arrhythmia was triggered by an undetected congenital birth defect. For this I am thankful—a hidden Atrial Septal Defect can be a big deal, and it often becomes one after it is too late.

The repair of this ASD can absolutely lead to further electrical (rhythm) problems. And for me, it certainly did.

Electrical problems can take many forms, and just like arrhythmia itself…it is all irregular.

When I was first stricken, I believe my naiveté was a blessing. In retrospect, I should have beelined to the hospital right away. But at that outset, my symptoms were not significant, nor certainly debilitating. I knew something was not right, but I also knew ("knew") that it was not a heart attack. I had no symptoms of heart attack or stroke. I had hoped it would pass, and really, I figured it was diet, stress or travel related. Thirty days of nonstop coffee I thought was a pretty significant event in its own right, and I figured my system was taking a few weeks to return to my daily rhythm of life, so to speak.

So I had no scope of context to communicate my light concern to the nice nurse at my primary care doctor's office. I was only moderately taken aback when she kindly suggested I go somewhere with the word "Emergency" over its door. When I did that, I had no concept of what to expect. I hadn't called my wife, I hadn't packed a bag, I hadn't made business preparations—I was blissfully faithful that a miracle of modern medicine would fix me up right then and there, and send me home. My one concern then was frankly, that they would take one quick look at my thirty-days-of-cake softened body, and mandate a strict diet. I also feared that they would loudly declare coffee verboten. I love coffee…and I really like cake, and when in Finland, I did my best to be a good guest at every sitting. I still thought coffee seventeen times a day was a swell concept, and I was eager to incorporate it into my American lifestyle (after all, I was young, strong, and in pretty good health—right?).

When they diagnosed classic Atrial Fibrillation in the Emergency Room, I took it as a temporary condition—especially as they could not pinpoint a cut and dried cause (nor cure). And in retrospect, I believe that was a time of yore when one could watch 30 minutes of television without seeing three ads for AFib-related drugs.

As it did not "go away" over the course of a few days, I became a little concerned, but also more curious.

Why was this happening to me?
How do I better protect my health?
Am I going to be crippled for the balance of my life?
How long might this life last?
Is this Cardioversion going to do significant harm?
Or any harm?
Will it affect my memory?
Is it safe?
Is it safe for me?

———

Upon that first Cardioversion, I figured I was out of the woods. It was a success, and while still groggy, I could feel my heart running smoothly and coolly underneath the surface.

When your heart beats normally, you don't notice it. It feels like a perfectly-tuned V6 motor—no roar and gurgle of a V8 exhaust, no rough ambition of a little four cylinder, no turbo lag—just smooth, quiet and consistent power there when you need it.

When one's heart is in arrhythmia of any form, there is nothing smooth about it. Erratic, stressed, irregular, and underpowered.

So coming back to Sinus rhythm, I felt like a new man!

But before I was released to a rewarding lunch, the doctors came with an assessment. I had a small hole in one chamber that was noticed by the TEE monitoring equipment. At the time I was strangely not concerned. I was clearly not yet completely sober. *But I saw the concern in Heather's eyes.*

The doctors were calm, and that helped my halcyon outlook. It was no emergency—nothing I had to take care of today, nor even really worry about. They wanted to watch it for a while. That's my kind of problem—I'll let you know if I feel any problems; otherwise I'll see you in about a year, and we can readdress it. I actually did not think it would warrant any further poking or prodding, or even electrocuting. I will eat better, I will not adopt my northern European caffeine diet, and I will exercise more strenuously—no problem. Youthful naiveté is a wonderful thing.

But as we digested the diagnosis for a few days, and especially as we recounted it to friends and family, I began to feel a little leery. And thankful. And frightened.

Then, of course I kept noticing and reading news stories about an otherwise healthy young guy dropping dead while playing basketball, taking a test in school, or just walking down the street.

So I began to feel even more thankful. Was I living on borrowed time? Had I cheated the odds to get this far? I was feeling fortunate, and a little nervous. And while it's always good to keep some gratitude deep in your heart, the nervousness about waiting for the other shoe to drop is not a comforting balance.

———

So, it's weird. How do I impart any advice, let alone any useful advice to the similarly afflicted? How do I offer any comfort while traversing the seven levels of frustration as they work to but cannot overcome this tiny yet pervasive lifestyle impediment?

All I can do is tell my story, in hopes that one might catch some similarities. And I will share what I have learned. Your story will be different, but some of the mechanics, so to speak, will be universal.

———

Communicate with your spouse and family. Even when you don't know the answer (and in my case, often even the question), talking it through can alleviate a lot of looming stress. It'll also help you bore down to the real questions and issues.

For a stoic, tough, independent-minded American with German roots, that is inherently difficult. And it's my heritage, Heather—it's not that I don't want to share, it's just that it is not in my DNA.

I had felt wonderfully at home in Finland, and not only because the Finns themselves were warm and welcoming. Part of it may have been that the land and climate is similar to my native Minnesota, where I hadn't lived for more than a decade. The other part may be best described in a joke that captures the Scandinavian sense of gregariousness. "How can you identify an outgoing Finn?" When he talks to you, he stares at your shoes instead of his own." That's me. Especially when faced with something I don't understand—I do not have an inherent desire to talk it through. I'll think about it, maybe even brood about it…and eventually make it my own and have my own plan of action.

In a complex (or even simple) medical situation—where friends and loved ones are potentially affected and are certainly concerned—that does not work. So I had to work at sounding things out. I owed that to Heather, at least, who is one of the world's great communicators. She does not always depress the clutch, which can make it tough for mere mortals to keep it up, but she does not keep anything bottled up.

I am particularly proud though that I did communicate well to my family, who is scattered across the country.

As I worked through the situation, I would update via email. I did so for two purposes; one to help the concepts gel in my mind, and two yes, to simply communicate any real technical information I learned. It's going to be less stressful on my mom in Florida if she can understand each step and technical points. Even, actually, if we do not understand the technicalities, when I can walk through a process it helps everyone's level of comfort.

I did so also to help my two younger brothers. As my dad has had a Pacemaker for more than two decades, and

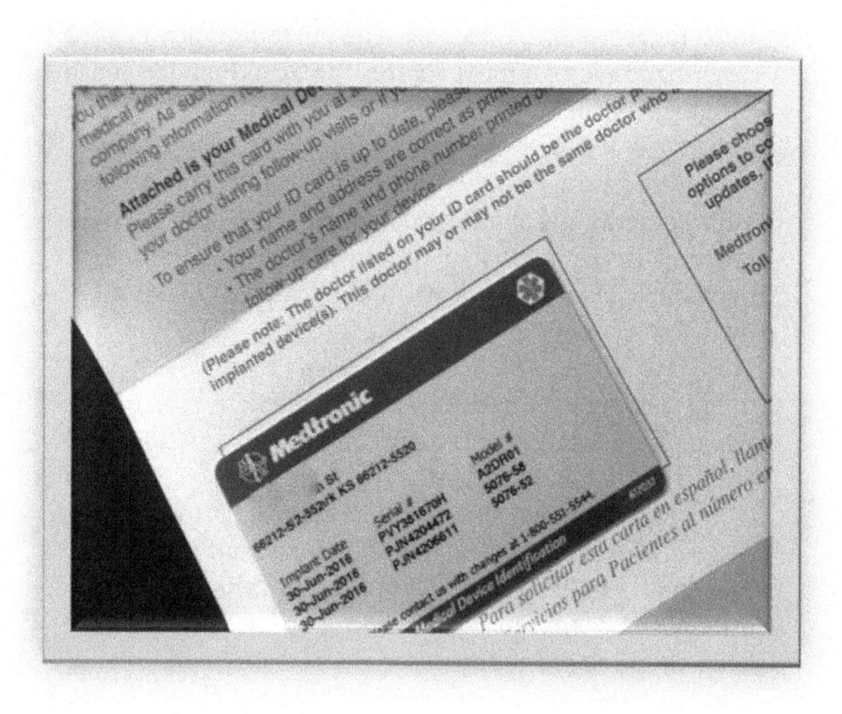

as part of my situation was congenital, I owed it to them to help share anything that might alleviate their concerns.

Even though I was young and truly invincible when my dad had become bionic, I still wondered—was this in my future?

I shared to my brothers that they in all likelihood had nothing about which to worry. My situation began because of the birth defect. Not totally uncommon, but also not life-threatening, and absolutely not something that is going to be fraternally consistent.

The Spouse's Perspective

WE'VE BOTH GAINED a great deal of perspective over these past recent years. Most of the newfound outlook of relativity is much-needed.

Our most recent trip to Mayo was cathartic in a number of ways. First, I was able to get over my two-month case of cancer. I do not mean to make light of it. There's nothing light about it—trust me—I carried that sucker on my shoulders and my psyche for sixty days. Life itself is tough. An unsolvable riddle within one's heart is frustrating. Adding the potential Big C on top of that is a quite a wallop.

The meeting with the urologists who granted my freedom opened the floodgates. Heather was beside herself. I was inappropriately stoic, on the outside. On the inside, I was counting—one down, one more to go. But absolutely, thank the Heavens for this small victory.

Beyond that, the cardiology sessions were almost lighthearted. And in fact, thanks to my new-est EP, the concluding meeting was. Just as all other Mayo professionals he spent enough time, answered questions, and really led a Socratic process to get *me* to the conclusion *I needed,* Dr. A was the same, and even better.

We talked through my multi-year history, and especially my recent goings-on. As I began spiraling myself into minutiae about daily routines, exercise levels, weight, stamina, heart rate ranges, hypothetical stimuli, and so on…and on, and on, he soon stopped me.

We went for a five-minute walk. Down the hall, up and down a few flights of stairs, and back to the examination room. My heart rate was fine. It accelerated a little bit with the light exertion, but perfectly normal. And especially normal for a forty-something guy in pretty good shape.

And then the appropriate sarcasm began. How was I able to take this walk without my GPS/heart rate watch? Did I get lost? Did I feel poorly? If I were not accompanied through the hospital halls by a highly trained physician, would I be able to find my way back?

"Your wife gave you that wonderful present (a shiny, non-GPS watch that she presented to me after we survived Maze surgery on my important "ticker")—that should be on your arm always! You do not need a silly heart rate monitor. If you feel poorly when you're out for a run, just slow down. Or stop. Or just go home. You're really in good shape, and, frankly, there is nothing more that medical science can do for you now.

Your obsession over statistics and tracking your progress is absolutely impeding your progress. What is our goal here? To get you back to living life as you'd like! Do that. Put that silly digital watch away, count your blessings, and count nothing more than that!"

I agreed with all the above, and was not antagonistic at all when I pointed out that I'm still on $300/month medications (to say nothing about my >30% annual insurance premium increase…). Dr. A calmly agreed that we would revisit that occasionally. If I progress okay, we can experiment taking me off them. In due time—nothing was to be fixed overnight, and I should know that by now. Duh….

Thank you for the good medical advice, and especially for putting my head in the right place with the good "life perspective" advice. Much more difficult to convey, but every bit as important as the nuts-and-bolts of medical science.

Our final-final session of that trip was with my "primary" cardiologist, Dr. N, and that session was similarly light and focused on big-picture, life issues. Do I notice any triggers, do I appreciate my daily routine, how do I adapt when out of routine? And then the whopper—do I get enough sleep?

I get six to seven hours of sleep on a regular basis. Some fluctuations are seasonal, and about once a month I am an incurable insomniac. But I don't let that bother me—I read through the night, and generally finally fall asleep about an hour before my normal morning time. I then plow through the day and sleep like a baby the next night. Strange, but strangely consistent, at least.

In a question-asking way, he got around to suggesting that I let myself sleep later. I responded that, as we had discussed ten minutes ago, waking early is a part of my daily routine that I really enjoy. And as much as I enjoy it, my dog and my wife like it even more. Heather's coffee is delivered upstairs, and Moxie has even more full-service benefit, no matter the weather.

As the good doctor went to far as to suggest that I go to sleep earlier, the conversation then devolved into a light-hearted marital counseling session. Two—thirds of our household would like to go to sleep earlier. But Heather's "quiet" time is when she is in bed but not yet ready to go to sleep. Therefore, *nobody* is ready to sleep. My doctor had a similar situation…and is no longer married. He did not go so far to suggest that we sleep in separate rooms or even anything more drastic, and it became a reminder that this is a two-way street. I am certain, though, that Dr. N was *on my side* as I described my silent 6:00 waking in stark contrast to Heather's midnight ramblings.

So we learn to get along, and we adapt, and try to appreciate those compromises. And I learn to take naps. I think I am constitutionally against the concept, but I began to appreciate the down time (and not feel guilty at wasting daylight), during my various recuperations. And now that I am "healthy," I aim to maintain that.

———

I say "we" a lot through this ordeal. I'm thankful, almost all of the time, to have a supportive, loving and pro-active spouse by my side. It can of course be tough when we look at things differently (frequently), but that's also a great backstop. Male/female stereotypes aside, it is invaluable to get another set of ears involved at each stop. Especially when what is between those ears is so sharp. I'll gladly take the minor battles over differences of interpretation when at the end of the day I know she is always advocating for me. Always.

And I try to remember that this is stressful on her, too. The tedious travel, the additional burden of daily chores, the lack of a 100% participatory partner each day, month, year is a drag. But the short-term concern and long-term worry is what's worst.

Heather recounted, with tears welling:

"I just needed you to feel better. I wondered what I could have done? I should have taken better care of you, and I felt like it was my job to know.

There was a general paranoia. I had no control over anything—nor did you—but I think in hindsight, knowledge would have been power. Although it's ludicrous now, what could I have done, what would I have done?

I got frustrated at times—not to the level that you did, because it was happening to you, not to me—but my frustration was driven when we were not getting the medical partnership, sympathy, empathy, that you deserved.

I know, I was annoying—I'm sorry. This was early on, when you'd been through several med changes, many cardioversions, and it felt like we were still experimenting—have they fixed it yet, have we fixed it yet? This was in part as we recalled my early significant recurrences. Heather, in full protective mode would regularly, often many times a day, ask me: "are you 'in fib,' are you okay?" After a while we changed that paradigm: I offered that I would simply, and always, tell her when I was 'in fib.' Otherwise, we could all assume that I was okay and in sinus rhythm.

I didn't know what to expect, no idea. And I wasn't going to form an opinion without any real information. I was clinging to hope, hope and more hope. I hoped we, and especially you, could learn to live with it. I hoped you could feel better. Even if this as always going to be an issue, I just needed you to feel better.

My panic and paranoia did decline, and we learned to live with it. Some of that was the good, responsive information we were getting from Mayo. And we learned to adapt, we did learn to live with it, and we did learn to accept it as a fact of life. Maybe, or rather, of course, getting used to it has made it easier to live with, and accept.

It was tough to think long-term; we were so narrowly-focused on the day to day, incident to incident, treatment to treatment. This process, each incident, was not 'one size fits all.' We had to deal with each day differently—this is today's scenario, this is the knowledge I have today, and have faith in our medical and personal daily decisions.

Some of my frustrations were because the provider often could not put themselves in our shoes! To them, it was the same old, same old. But each of those "same old" cases happens to be a real person, a real patient, hopeful, every day, to feel better.

While working with these providers, it felt like we had to be proactive, patient and relentless. It was funny, we were trying to consume all the information we could, while also being a little bit patient. We needed to take it all in, filter it, augment with the Internet and filter that even more. We're trying to educate ourselves, but it really became a matter of identifying what we could control, and in the same breath, accepting what we could not control—and that was most of it.

We had to intermittently share frustration, anger, impatience and thankfulness. And on a regular basis, we had to re-remind ourselves that modern medicine has not yet cracked this one. And while simple Atrial Fibrillation affects more than 25% of the mature population, in the grand scheme of things, this is not tremendously critical.

We were pretty good at reminding ourselves to not resign to 'this is the best I'm going to get.' When it was always changing, we were pretty good at following a path, pursuing something different, and trying again.

But it was always frustrating.

A Mother's Perspective

THERE'S A SAYING among mothers...you're only as happy as your least happy child. This applies to healthy also, because if a child of mine is struggling with a health issue, I'm not only unhappy for him, I'm worried and frightened.

Most kids' health issues are relatively mild and easily remedied, but when an adult child has an ongoing issue with his heart, there is not much peace in my heart. Since I don't live near Adam, I don't see him often, but we talk, and he has done a remarkable job of keeping me informed as things change, improve, un-improve, regress, digress, complicate and confuse. And as he undergoes seemingly endless tests, changes of medications and procedure after procedure after procedure.

Adam had a bad episode of AFib while he was in Florida a few years ago, (not his first) and had to go back to Kansas earlier than originally planned. I picked him up in Sarasota to drive him to the Tampa airport. My beautiful, strong, tall, healthy son, of whom I have always been so proud, and loved with all my heart, had a gray complexion, was visibly weak and shaky. What's a mother to do? Drive him to the airport, of course, with hands clenched on the steering wheel, barely able to breathe, trying to act like this was a normal trip to the airport. When we got there, he asked for a wheelchair and one was provided. We said goodbye and as the gentleman prepared to wheel him to the gate, he leaned over to me, put a hand on my shoulder and said "don't worry, we'll take care of him." Where would we be without the kindness of strangers?

I managed to drive myself back home safely without a major meltdown, with updates coming regularly from Adam as he made his way throughout the airport, onto his plane, and ultimately delivered safely into the arms of his wife.

Of course, then came more tests, different drugs, different procedures. Some worked for a while and then didn't. Bringing us to the summer of "the mother of all heart surgeries." We were all outwardly calm as we gathered in Rochester MN at the Mayo Clinic, where the "best heart surgeon in the world" plies his craft. We head to the hospital before the crack of dawn, they take him away and Heather and I calmly (hah!) wait in the designated waiting area and hospital staff keep us updated. "He is on heart/lung bypass now." I definitely did not need to know that. A short time later, " he is off by-pass now." I definitely did need to know that.

My worst moment came, oddly, as we approached his room in ICU. Sedated, sleeping, whatever, tubes and wires and beepers and ringers and tappers and clangers, and that "unconscious" demeanor. I guess because he was unconscious. I stopped in my tracks with tears in my eyes and shaking hands. Really wanted to back up for a moment to re-group when his nurse Glenn (sometimes known as Saint Glenn) greeted us, introduced himself and gave us no time to be afraid. He calmly told us what was going on, what to expect and shared his own experience of heart surgery at the hands of "the best surgeon in the world." He even showed us his scar! He suggested this might be a good time to get something to eat as Adam would sleep for a while. We did. I actually was able to eat something, I think. When we returned, Glenn had removed the dreadful tube that was in Adam's throat. What an improvement! At least in my ability to deal with this.

Time passed, we all went home, Adam recovered from the surgery, not an easy process, but the heart began to mis-behave again. His, that is. Mine is breaking for him. More tests, different drugs and another trip to Mayo a year later. Now a pacemaker, a much easier procedure and it's looking like we have found a solution.

Through all of my own fear, worry, concern, the thousands of emotions that we all go through when someone we love is struggling, I never once doubted that there was an answer for him, and that he would find it, his heart would behave and he could continue the healthy productive life he deserves.

I guess that's what a mother's heart does. It believes.

Conclusion

THERE IS HOPE!

Of course there is, but today I am describing Honest-to-God, genuine scientific hope. This layman is eager to report that the experts are considering the patients' perspective in treatment.

The science is important. But to each patient, the polestar is: "how does this help me?" *How does it feel, what is the effect...how does it affect my life?*

Cue the Scandinavians! I am pleased to recommend that you read this research article: **"Patients' Experiences of Living with Atrial Fibrillation: A Mixed Methods Study."**

Marie Stridsman, 1 Anna Stro¨mberg, 2,3 Jeroen Hendriks, 2,4 and Ulla Walfridsson, 2,3

1 Feelgood Fo¨retagsha¨lsa, Linko¨ping, Sweden
2 Department of Medical and Health Sciences, Division of Nursing, Linko¨ping University, Linko¨ping, Sweden

3 Department of Cardiology, Link¨oping University Hospital, Link¨oping, Sweden
4 Centre for Heart Rhythm Disorders, University of Adelaide,
South Australian Health & Medical Research Institute and Royal Adelaide Hospital, Adelaide, Australia

Correspondence should be addressed to Ulla Walfridsson; ulla.walfridsson@regionostergotland.se
Received 28 April 2019; Revised 24 September 2019; Accepted 26 October 2019; Published 3 December 2019
Academic Editor: Elena Cavarretta

Reading this recent analysis was heart-warming for yours truly.

The *Introduction* states: "Awareness of epidemiological and clinical consequences of atrial fibrillation (AF) has increased, as have disease-related costs. Less attention has been paid to patient-related issues, such as understanding how symptoms, different therapies, and lifestyle adjustments affect daily life. We aimed to describe patients' experience of living with AF."

Once more, with emphasis: "We aimed to describe patients' *experience of living with AF!"* That's gold. Every italicized word is important. Nothing is solved, but I am thrilled to read of the researchers' emphasis on the patient experience. And how the patient *lives with* AFib.

In addition to quantitative data, patients completed questionnaires on: symptoms, health-related quality of life (HRQOL), depression, anxiety and perceived control. Sound familiar?

The mixed-method study drew correlations between the physiological effects of AFib with the real-life ramifications upon the patient. I am glad for the reinforcement. Generally speaking, patients' biggest life impact was concern for role limitations due to physical health problems and (lessened) vitality.

"Fatigue was described as a 'constant companion.' Not being physically active resulted in weight gain for some patients. Patients described that they needed to rest more, avoided tiring activities, and had to reduce their pace of activities."

"Patients expressed feeling that they were in an unusual situation by being dependent upon others for housework, gardening, and driving longer distances. Due to their lack of energy, they were unable to work and withdrew from other people and social activities. '*I withdrew, wanted to be alone, and could not cope with being around other people.*'"

"The limitations were also mental. Not being able to perform usual activities during AF caused restlessness accompanied with frustration. Feeling tired affected the patients' mood. They became increasingly irritated, which had a negative effect on their social lives. '*You become like a child, a bit fussy when you are tired.*'"

"One patient described the inability to concentrate on something else other than the symptoms of AF: '*When you only focus on atrial fibrillation, you get nothing else done.'"*

"Never knowing when the next episode might occur led to an unsecure living situation with a constant feeling of worry for both patients and families. *'You become limited, restricted, and do not participate, you say no and do not do things you would like to do.' 'You worry about practical aspects of having a relapse of AF, how to get home and where to leave the kids.'"*

"Patients stated that the first experience of AF was very frightening, especially before being diagnosed and receiving an explanation about what they experienced. *'The first time I had it, I was really worried. I hardly dared to fall asleep because I thought I might never wake up again.'"*

"Repeated AF episodes caused a lot of distress. Patients worried about long-term effects and feared the infliction of serious damage to the heart. *'You only have one heart.'"*

"Other worries were fear of adverse drug reactions.... *'Oh my God, am I going to take those damn medicines for the rest of my life? It could certainly not be good at all.'"*

"It was difficult for respondents to reconcile themselves to being patients, and it was common to feel that it was "unfair" and "scary" to be young and have AF. *'My wife is very worried, but she does not dare show it because that makes me worried.'* Some patients avoided mentioning recurrences to not worry family members. Family members' behavior could cause annoyance. Patients could get irritated due to repeated questions such as "how do you feel" or due to relatives taking their pulse."

———

If you've had a family member touched by AFib—even asymptomatic arrhythmia—you are familiar with many of these concepts.

The study's *Conclusion* cites: "The mixed methods design deepens our understanding of challenges faced by patients. Patients experienced a limited ability to perform activities of daily living due to AF which created different kinds of worries that encouraged the use of various strategies to manage their lives. Healthcare providers need to be aware that relationships between patients and their relatives can change, and therefore they need to be supported and integrated into the care system."

Hallelujah.

———

My saga has dragged on long enough. At least this chapter of my life. Thank you for reading. I'm going to try to quit complaining now. And not let it define me or bog me down.

Thank you, my friend, for your sagacity throughout, and especially in review:

"I think you should 'thrive with it.'

You are missing a very important point. Atrial fibrillation actually saved your life from even more misery. It might even be possible to think of it as a friendly arrhythmia, at least someday,

AFib led to the echocardiogram which led to the most important diagnosis - atrial septal defect. You cannot thrive with an atrial septal defect, especially once the shunting results in Eisenmenger's Syndrome.

Your main, and most important diagnosis, has been made and corrected."

Good perspective.

And thank you to all dedicated providers, and especially to my lovely, patient and pro-active wife. It's been tough on us both—to say nothing of how I've tried the dog's patience. I know it's been tough on those close to me. Particularly on parents, for whom that noun is also a verb that never ceases. Thank you, Mom and Dad, for your support, but I've got this one.

It's tough, and while it is not totally life-threatening, it is a lifestyle-impingement. But in my case, this several-year saga of frustration has saved my life. Twice, at least.

Head up. Do what you can. Be pro-active. Every day. Live with it. Love with it. Thrive with it. Be thankful for the ability to function with it. Run with it.

Be competitive with it. Don't be ashamed to take a nap because of it. Maintain perspective because of it. Thank loved ones because of it. Enjoy each sunrise because of it.

LIVE with it!

And don't be so frustrated—your case is likely simpler than mine.

Postscript: Iatrogenic, Doc

YOUR OVER-HUMBLED *scribe was "in lockup." A third time dofetilide initiation. That is nine total days of immobility, going on nearly 1,500 days into my arrhythmic saga.*

My text-message conversant is a terrific childhood friend. Despite our best attempts to kill each other during years of teenage invincibility, he is now a cardiologist. A great one, with a concise and down-to-earth perspective, perhaps enhanced by several states' worth of distance from me…and a couple decades of maturity.

———

Kind of a goat-schtup over here. Took me off Diltiazem because my rate is down in the low 50s. Rhythm, though, seems to move between AFib, and "sinus arrhythmia." No real plan other than: "Well, we hope the Tikosyn will work."

Premature confusion (but after 48 hours of no direction/communication). Good talk with Dr. J—I've not known him until meeting while he's on hospital rounds this weekend. Sinus arrhythmia is okay/good. AFib was misinterpreted. Confident in Tikosyn. Discharge in 24 hours (it is now 1:37 pm). No zap to be necessary.

I think Dr. J is the author of a very famous book in the industry. I haven't seen any of your tracings but I'm very confident that dofetilide will work.

He recommended another book to me, referencing all-around wellness. He thinks my problems are exacerbated by exercise, and wants me to do less. And do yoga (HA!). But I do feel better after that conversation.

You know that you're a total dork when Siri autocompletes dofetilide for you.

You're a good doctor when Siri recognizes those words. I'm a chronic patient because my phone does. Ugh.

I think yoga is one of the best ideas I've heard. Or whatever method helps you find your center and calm it down. I know I've never been able to.

You should seriously write a book about this from the patient's perspective. I know a lot of patients who would want to read about your experience.

Think of all the work you could get done during dofetilide initiations.

That's not a bad idea, thanks. Except that it's tough to get work done while locked up. No sleep—poking and prodding around the clock. Nothing to make a guy feel bad like spending time in a hospital.

Tell me about it. Imagine how I feel.

You get to walk around in fancy suits and tell people what to do. Sitting and waiting...and not being able to punch the third-string blood-sucker when she shuffles in and slams on the light and smacks her purple bubble gum at two am is another story.

I'll think about yoga. It may not be a bad idea, but I'm having trouble shifting my paradigm—I have gone through all this rigmarole so that I could get back to the lifestyle I like, including exercise (which, I thought, was also preventative). He's essentially saying I should take it easier, and do about half what I've normally done.

Irony. Now you've got a great book.

You could come at it from a less is more argument. I'd gladly write a chapter about less being more in medicine.

Short chapter!

You do have me thinking, though. I'll give it some more, earnest thought.

Chapter three: Siri can auto-complete dofetilide, but not rigmarole.

Touché!

You should. I'm serious. Atrial fib is a massive problem and we don't do a good job with it. There are all sorts of books describing medicine and science, but I'm not aware of anything that describes the pain in the ass, both from a patient and physician perspective.

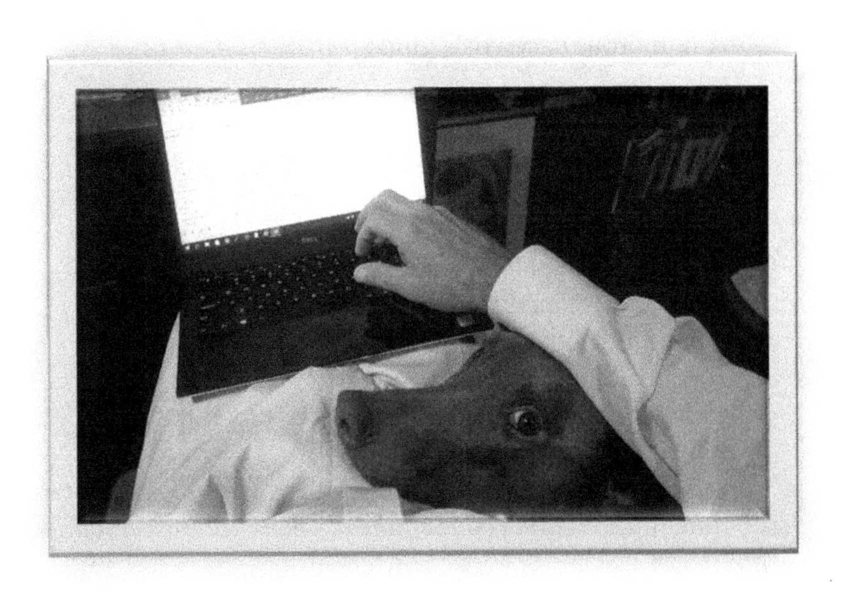

I guess you have been listening to my travails over the years. It is a pain in the ass, and it is frustrating. I hadn't considered how "troubling" it might be, from a physician's perspective, to not be able to give straight-line advice...or just fix the damned thing.

You would have millions of potential readers.

You do have me thinking. And it could be fun. At first blush, though, I can't see any clear, useful direction...other than the solution-less pain in the ass.

Make it funny.

Yeah, it's real funny, asshole. Funny as a crutch.

A humorous survivor's guide.

I guess there is some humor in the perpetual futility. Sometimes tough for me to remember that, though. I will try.

I'll let you in on a secret. Electrophysiology is a controversial specialty within our profession. I would like nothing more than to see a practical, intelligent person make a joke out of the way atrial fib is traditionally "managed." Because it is a total joke. My opinion.

And with a shared sentiment from a respected physician....

I'm inclined to agree. It's a crap shoot—except all other guys throw up their hands and say "that's the EP's department." All other doctors are eager to distance themselves from arrhythmia conversation/questions.

My ten minutes with Dr. J was the most comprehensive, yet still head-scratching conversation I've had about it (this time around) with anyone other than you.

I just about got in a fistfight with one last week. I'm kind of done.

And quite often, their treatments suck.

I agree. A ground-level example is that Heather has been waiting since Thursday for a call back directly. Frustrating, as we get three (at least!) different opinions each day here. She's hoping he can be a one-stop clearinghouse for her questions.

Dr. J did offer to me: "Adam, with your situation, you can ask ten different cardiologists, and get 11 different opinions." This was, however, after he said he did speak with my EP this morning by phone.

I'm at the gym now, about to exercise. I'm all worked up. It sure would be ironic if I went into atrial fib.

Lucky you! I'm watching KU/OU basketball. Another spectacular game. And I'm thinking of making notes/outline of this saga.

Glad to hear. I'm in sinus tach.

Iatrogenic.

Thank you for teaching me a new word. Maybe a book title right there....

It's a great word that I (unfortunately) use frequently at work.

This is not a good sign....

CPSIA information can be obtained
at www.ICGtesting.com
Printed in the USA
LVHW050848261121
704455LV00008B/908